Spirituality

Reiki Healing Guide on How to Improve Your Health and Positive Energy

(Healing Yourself With Crystals, Opening Your Third Eye and Connecting With Universal Energy With Yoga)

Llyn Honervogt

Published by Rob Miles

Llyn Honervogt

All Rights Reserved

Spirituality: Reiki Healing Guide on How to Improve Your Health and Positive Energy (Healing Yourself With Crystals, Opening Your Third Eye and Connecting With Universal Energy With Yoga)

ISBN 978-1-989990-49-0

All rights reserved. No part of this guide may be reproduced in any form without permission in writing from the publisher except in the case of brief quotations embodied in critical articles or reviews.

Legal & Disclaimer

The information contained in this book is not designed to replace or take the place of any form of medicine or professional medical advice. The information in this book has been provided for educational and entertainment purposes only.

The information contained in this book has been compiled from sources deemed reliable, and it is accurate to the best of the Author's knowledge; however, the Author cannot guarantee its accuracy and validity and cannot be held liable for any errors or omissions. Changes are periodically made to this book. You must consult your doctor or get professional medical advice before using any of the suggested remedies, techniques, or information in this book.

Upon using the information contained in this book, you agree to hold harmless the Author from and against any damages, costs, and expenses, including any legal fees potentially resulting from the application of any of the information provided by this guide. This disclaimer applies to any damages or injury caused by the use and application, whether directly or indirectly, of any advice or information presented, whether for breach of contract, tort, negligence, personal injury, criminal intent, or under any other cause of action.

You agree to accept all risks of using the information presented inside this book. You need to consult a professional medical practitioner in order to ensure you are both able and healthy enough to participate in this program.

Table of Contents

INTRODUCTION 1

CHAPTER 1: WHAT ARE CHAKRAS? 5

CHAPTER 2: MEANING OF YOGA 11

CHAPTER 3: HANDS ON SELF-TREATMENT ROUTINE 15

CHAPTER 4: REIKI HEALING ART VARIES AMONG INDIVIDUAL PRACTITIONERS 24

CHAPTER 5: CRYSTAL/PYRAMID AND ITS TREATMENT METHODS 32

CHAPTER 6: THE SECOND CHAKRA 50

CHAPTER 7: THE DIFFERENCE BETWEEN REIKI AND ANGELIC REIKI 56

CHAPTER 8: REIKI TIPS FOR BEGINNERS 63

CHAPTER 9: HEALTH BENEFITS OF REIKI 69

CHAPTER 10: MAINTAINING THE VIBRATION OF A HEALER IN THE FACE OF DAILY LIFE 76

- CHAPTER 11: KARMA/BLOCKAGES ... 88
- CHAPTER 12: TREATING OTHERS WITH REIKI ... 98
- CHAPTER 13: EXERCISES FOR SPECIFIC AREAS OF THE BODY ... 105
- CHAPTER 14: LIVING WITH AN ATTITUDE OF GRATITUDE ... 111
- CHAPTER 15: REIKI FOR STRESS RELIEF ... 125
- CHAPTER 16: A SIMPLE MEDITATION. ... 137
- CHAPTER 17: MORE ADVANTAGES OF REIKI ... 140
- CHAPTER 18: ENERGETICBODIES ... 144
- CHAPTER 19: ATTUNEMENT - ALL DEGREES ... 166
- CHAPTER 20: MEDITATION ... 181
- CONCLUSION ... 188

Introduction

There are plenty of books on this subject on the market, thanks again for choosing this one! Every effort was made to ensure it is full of as much useful information as possible, please enjoy!

What Is Reiki?

Its operation is based on releasing and regulating the flow of Ki in the body. The Ki - for the Chinese Chi and Prana for the Hindus - is the force that is ultimately responsible for constituting and giving life to the matter that makes up our body. A free and abundant flow of Ki guarantees us an optimum level of health. Under these same parameters, other therapies such as acupuncture, shiatsu and various types of massage work. However, Reiki

Ryoho offers us something more important than this.

The founder of the system, the Japanese Mikao Usui, studied and practiced various systems of meditation and inner development. People who learned the system with Usui, in addition to the various therapeutic techniques, learned to practice meditation and Kiko - Chi kung in Chinese - as well as teachings about different forms of spirituality, in order to promote balance and inner growth of the practitioners

Thus, Reiki Ryoho, besides being a therapy, is also a spiritual practice. In the same way as meditation, prayer or any system of inner growth, Reiki Ryoho is practiced by people of all kinds of creeds in the world and including those who do not manifest a definite faith.

The spirit is part of the nature of the human being and spiritual maturation is another phase of the process of the natural evolution of the person. The different forms of spirituality are only a support for this process, just as sport is for physical development and education for the intellectual.

The maturation of the person is not complete as long as their spiritual maturation process is not performed. As in the physical and mental levels, each person has their own rhythm of maturation. The strength and stability of the spirit is another factor within the level of health of the person. The spirit relies on the mind, emotions, and body for its stability. A firm spirit is a sign of good health in general. A good connection with the spirit does not provide the guidance and sensitivity necessary to maintain balance in our body and emotions.

Reiki Ryoho, practiced in the way it was conceived, is a system to balance not only the body but also the psyche and the soul. In short, Reiki therapy is a discipline that seeks the growth and strengthening of the person at all levels, promoting the balance, freedom, and fulfillment of each individual.

Under these premises, this book is presented. This book is intended to provide the reader with foundations of theoretical, practical and attitudinal knowledge on which the growth process itself can be based.

Chapter 1: What Are Chakras?

There are various vibration levels that surround the human body and within the body there are different energy centers which connect different glands and organs. These energy centers are known as chakras, which in Sanskrit means "wheel". Therefore, a chakra is a wheel-like vortex which moves in a circular motion and forms a vacuum at the center. This vacuum then attracts anything near it as long as it is within its vibratory level. There are actually a lot of chakras in the body. As these chakras attract coded information around them, they also radiate vibration energy.

The 7 main chakras in the body are connected to the human being on spiritual, mental, emotional, and physical levels. Each chakra has a physical main gland or organ which resonate a frequency. As an illustration, the heart chakra is connected to the heart organ, thymus gland, immune system, hands, arms, secondary circulatory system, lymph glands, immune system, bronchia system, and lungs. It is responsible for their functioning. Green is the color of the heart chakra.

These chakra centers are found along the spinal column. If there is any disturbance on any of the chakra, it will show in its vitality level. Furthermore, each of the chakra has its own intelligence center. Therefore, the chakra isn't only connected to a person's physical health but also to the belief, mental, and emotional systems. It is imperative to keep each chakra balanced in order for the body to function effectively. The chakra vibrations must be able to vibrate the same frequency.

If a chakra is out of balance, it is possible that it will also affect the neighboring chakras and the other parts of the body. An out of balance chakra can mean that it is blocked, congested, under-active, or over-active. It will manifest and be felt by you on a physical, emotional, or mental level.

Why Energies Affect the Chakras

Sunlight is the main provider of energy, heat, and light. It sustains not only the life on Earth but also Earth itself. Through photosynthesis, plants are supplied with energy to sustain the lives of you, me, and even animals. Sunlight has electromagnetic waves, which also includes long and short radio waves, microwaves, infrared rays, visible light rays, x-rays, gamma rays, and cosmic rays. These energies are used by all human beings in their daily lives. However, not much emphasis is put on visible light rays, which can break down into various beams of colors if a prism is used towards the sun. This visible light is broken down into seven color energies, namely, violet, indigo, blue, green, yellow, orange, and red. It is actually the colors of the rainbow.

Each color has its own vibration frequency and wavelength. Thus, each color has a different effect on the individual. The color red has the slowest frequent and the longest wavelength which people recognize as stimulating and warm. The color violet has the fastest frequency and shortest wavelength. It is recognized by people as calming and cool. The eyes receive the color and light information. These impulses, which pass through the optic nerve to the brain through the pituitary gland, can trigger secretion of hormones to the different parts of the body. A lot of functions of the body can be depressed or stimulated by the various light colors and, which in turn, affect the chakras.

Because colors and light affect the hormones and glands, they also influence the feelings and moods of a person. In fact, science has proven that there are colors which stimulate mental activity while there are also colors which calm the mind. Light energy nourishes the brain, the physical body, the emotions, and the chakras. The extra color energy can also be received from color bathing, deco, clothing, minerals, sound, aromatherapy, vitamins, herbs, and colored foods.

Why Are Chakras Important

Toxins and other impurities have been proven by medical science to have an influence on the human body. In fact, poor environmental factors, chemicals in foods, and negative thoughts can also cause imbalances in the chakra system, which can manifest on the physical level. Because traditional health care can't cure or alleviate the symptoms, you and I must strive to seek ways to improve our health.

By understanding the chakra system, we can harmonize the spirit, mind, and body by ensuring that each of the chakra centers is working with each other. The optimum health is achieved if the mental, physical, spiritual, and emotional parts are all strong. Each of us must emphasize not only independence but interdependence as well. Each of the chakras is interdependent to achieve balance and harmony.

Chapter 2: Meaning Of Yoga

The word "yoga" has a Sanskrit origin, which means to join the physical body with the inner soul. Yoga is a practice that, through specific body postures and breathing techniques, ultimately aims to achieve health and relaxation.

Reasons to practice yoga

There are a lot of reasons to practice yoga, and the reasons may vary for each individual. However, the most common and sensible reasons include but are not limited to:

Stress relief

Relief from pain

Better breathing and circulation

Flexibility and agility of body

Increase in strength

Weight management

Improved blood circulation in body

Cardiovascular advantages

Focus and concentration

Inner peace

Pre-requisites to practicing yoga

Practice yoga daily for about 30-45 minutes.

Early morning is the perfect time to perform yoga. However, you can even do it in the afternoon, provided the food restrictions are taken care of.

It is ideal to do yoga on an empty stomach. If you are performing it in the afternoon, you should not consume any liquid or solid for an hour or two before your yoga session.

For children below 12, the duration of yoga should be minimal. It is better not to overstretch or overdo any asana, without consulting experts.

Yoga cannot be performed on bare ground. It should be done either on a carpet or a mat.

Choose a bright, spacious, clean and airy place to perform yoga.

Yoga should be practiced wearing comfortable clothes.

Diet and yoga go hand in hand. It is better to avoid hot and spicy food for better results of yoga.

Vegetarian diet is generally agreed to be the best combination with yoga.

Women should avoid yoga during pregnancy and menstrual cycles.

Do not push yourself too much doing a particular pose or asana. If you are not comfortable, just skip and go ahead.

To do all the asana and poses, one should be first mentally prepared to take the strain and challenge.

Chapter 3: Hands On Self-Treatment Routine

Reiki self-hands on therapy is an **energy booster**, with **unlimited potential**, always available and accessible when you need it; it starts gently and instantly whenever and wherever you place your hands on your body, and in the process, it balances body's energy field and all the chakras, aka the energy centers. The automatic Reiki energy flow comes directly from your hands to your cells; in turn, your cells are rejuvenating from this energy. This can be compared with a weak battery that requires **energy** to be recharged.

The more you use Reiki hands on positions, the more you become attuned to it. Before practicing Reiki, make sure that you are in a very calm state of mind to fully enjoy its benefits. The "heat" generated through the palms releases endorphins that act as pain inhibitors.

By simply placing the hands over your body, Reiki energy starts flowing automatically. One day soon, you'll start feeling a very strong inner peace, a pure joy, some sort of message coming from the **Source**. At that precise moment you'll know that something out of the ordinary is taking place. Reiki's purpose is to **assist the body's natural healing process**. This open hands on technique will help you understand the real Reiki, the one and only that was used by our ancestors.

If you are not feeling the energy flow when self-treating, it is normal and there is nothing to worry about. Remember to always keep your hands slightly cupped with all the fingers together. You always have few minutes throughout the day when you can place your hands on yourself and let Reiki flow. Do this as often as you can, whenever you think about it; it will soon become **second nature** to you, and keep doing it on a daily basis.

Please always remember to use your intuition, it knows best! Always keep a couple of pillows or foam blocks (like the one we use in yoga) handy when your arms or wrists get tired (just squeeze a pillow under them).

To calm you down: one hand on the back of your head and the other hand on the Third Eye.

Fear: 1 drop of Tee Tree oil on your Solar Plexus with one hand on the top of it, and the other hand in the back of your head.

Headaches & Migraines: Lavender is again the mother of relief. Put a couple of Lavender oils in your palms. Lay them down to the part of the head where the pain is most severe, and then put both hands on your temples, on your hears and then on your Solar Plexus. Migraine being usually a chronic condition, you can also treat your neck and shoulders areas as well.

The Hands on Positions

Keep your hands for at least 3 minutes for each position. You will start with a 3 minute session and then after a couple of weeks, set up your reiki timer to 5 minutes, and so on.

The head positions

H1 Both hands together cover the eyes. It is a good position for the third Eye chakra that facilitates meditation. The entire body is reflected in the face.

H2 Put your hands to the right and left of your temples. Good for stress, tiredness, headache, pituitary gland, immune defense and hormone imbalances. It also treats the nerves, including mental and emotional problems, concentration etc.

H3 Both hands cupped on each side of the head, covering the ears. Good for your ears, nose and throat problems, colds, balance, hearing.

H4 Both hands are behind the head, like a "bowl", and cover the back of your head. Good for stress, worry, headache; Colds, including brain, neck and back problems, spinal nerve problems.

H5 Both hands cover the top of the head aka the "Crown Chakra". It is where the human being connects with the universe. This Chakra is connected to the unification of the higher self with the personality, illumination, universal consciousness and a higher knowing. It governs the pineal gland, cerebral cortex and the central nervous system.

The body positions

B1 Hold hands and fingers so they form a "tent" around the throat. This Chakra is connected to communication, voicing your thoughts and feelings, your desires and dislikes, the freedom to express yourself and the power to make changes. It governs the throat, thyroid, para-thyroid, larynx, mouth, tongue, neck and shoulders.

B2 Solar plexus and Heart position. Breast position. It is good for the 4th Chakra. Heart, thymus, lungs, asthma, allergies, circulation problems, immune system, emotional problems etc.

B3 Solar plexus position, under the breasts and over the lower ribs. It is good for the 3rd Chakra. The sternum system, lungs, pancreas, liver, spleen, gallbladder. Digestive problems, stress, worry, nervousness, control, etc.

B4 Place the hands approximately around the liver area. It is good for the 2nd

Chackra. Digestive organs, liver, spleen, gallbladder, kidneys, adrenal gland. Depression, emptiness, disability to feel happiness.

B5 Hands by the pubic bone. Angle your hands so they follow the groin. It is good for the 1st and 2nd Chakras. Reproduction system, testicles, ovaries, kidneys, adrenal glands, urinary problems. Tiredness, weight problems, sexual problems, physical and emotional.

The Back positions

BA1 Hands over the shoulder blades. Treating neck and shoulders, heart area, protective instinct, and depression. Stress and headaches, along with responsibility problems.

BA2 Hands approximately at the middle of the back above the kidneys. Treating stress, allergies, relationship problems.

Heart and lung area, kidneys, adrenal glands, lymph and diaphragm.

BA3 Lower back, below the waist. Treating Chakra 1, pelvic area, reproductive system, digestive system etc. Relationship and emotional problems.

The legs and feet positions

L1 Kneecaps, place one hand above the kneecap and one hand under the knee. Treat each knee separately. It is good for knee injuries, disability to bend (mentally). Headache, stiffness in the neck. Energy blockage in the lower body.

L2 Ankles, do each one separately. Hold your hands in the position most comfortable for you. It is good for energy blockages, problems with neck and throat, thyroid gland and lymph. You can also treat each foot separately. One hand should cover the sole of the foot, otherwise hold in the most comfortable position for you. The feet contain reflex zones for all the organs in the body. All the organs and chakras will be treated.

Chapter 4: Reiki Healing Art Varies Among Individual Practitioners

The different techniques of Reiki healing art can be as unique as the individuals who practice them. There are no hard and fast rules to Reiki energy healing, although some Masters claim that their way is "best". You can learn all of the different techniques that you want, but you are the one who decides what is "right" for you.

One Master tells a story about visiting another practitioner who used crystals and it did not "feel" right to her. Crystals can be empowered with the energy that is Reiki. They can be part of Reiki healing art. But, they are only necessary if the practitioner "feels" they are necessary.

Symbols, signs, specific hand positions and movements may all be used during a Reiki energy healing. Or, a practitioner may use only his mind to heal himself or another. The real power does not lie in the "props" that we use to heal. The real power lies within us and around us.

Anyone can learn the Reiki healing art. All it takes is acceptance of and understanding of the infinite energy that is called Reiki by some, but has many different names in many different cultures.

Learning the Reiki healing art, just as with any art form, is a journey. You follow a path as long as you feel that you are going in the right direction. It is possible to become lost, but if you allow your own intuition to be your guide, you will eventually find your way.

You may need to read different viewpoints, attend different classes or visit different practitioners. You may need to do your own research. Some Masters have found that their journeys led them to

Japan, where they could see and "feel" the places where the practice originated.

But, it is not necessary to travel or attend seminars to begin to use Reiki energy healing in your own life. You can learn all that you need to know from a book or through a video, in the comfort of your own home, at your own pace. If you feel that you want more knowledge, you can attend classes or travel the world. The choice is yours.

You may become discouraged on your journey, but don't give up. Particularly if you are discouraged because another "Master" tells you that you are "wrong" or the way you have learned is wrong. If it is "right" for you, it is right.

"Every Master that you meet, is simply a Master of their own path to enlightenment," is a quote from the book Radical Reiki, Radical Life. They may have studied for years and be proficient in the

Reiki healing art, but their power is no greater than your own.

The Reiki Healing Touch FAQ

Reiki is often misunderstood by the mainstream media and public opinion. Seen as a hoax or even witchcraft and an opening into devil worship! Misinformation and poor understanding of Reiki has led to many myths developing so I thought I would but down a simple FAQ about the main aspects of Reiki to help bring a clearer picture to the art.

Q. "What is Reiki?"

A. Reiki is originally a Japanese art of energy healing which promotes stress reduction and relaxation that promotes self healing. It is typically administered by laying hands on a person to allow life force energy to flow into the subject. Boosting this energy helps us by being happier and healthier which can counter illness.

Q. "What does it feel like?"

A. Reiki treatment has been described as sensations of heat or coolness, "pins and needles" tingling, vibrational buzzing, electrical sparks, throbbing, numbness, itchiness and even drowsiness.

Q. "Is Reiki a religion?"

A. No! Reiki is not a religion. While spiritual in nature Reiki does not have any dogma or churches or anything of the sort. It is also not linked to faith healing or witchcraft. It can be seen as a very personal spiritual thing and many have attributed it to feeling closer to god if they are religious but the foundations of Reiki are not religious in nature. Reiki will in fact work whether you believe in it or not!

Q. "Is Reiki dangerous?"

A. Reiki is not an intrusive treatment but one that promotes the body to heal itself. In this way it is believed to be very safe as there are no external chemicals like medicine and no surgery. Just energy flow that removes blockages from the body and promotes self healing that the body knows how to do!

Q. "Where does this energy come from?"

A. The energy that flows from Reiki does not come from the Reiki practitioner not from the patient. The energy comes from the universe and has an infinite supply.

Q. "Can I treat myself with Reiki?"

A. Yes you can! This is a great asset of Reiki that you can use the same treatment of others on yourself to promote your own health.

Q. "Can anyone learn Reiki?"

A. Again Yes! Reiki can be learned by anyone. Adult, child, male, female, skeptic and believer Reiki can be taught to anyone you do not need any prerequisite talent or initiation.

Q. "Can I stop going to the doctor if I use Reiki?"

A. Reiki works in conjunction with all other medicine and most Reiki practitioners do not recommend that you stop using conventional medical advice in favor of Reiki only. Reiki can be used along side all other treatments for tremendous benefit.

Q. "What are Reiki Symbols?"

A. The Reiki symbols are simply tools to use as focus points.

Q. "Can Reiki be used at a distance?"

A. Yes, at a higher level of Reiki you can send energy to anyone at any distance.

You need to have a picture of the person or their name on a piece of paper and use one of the symbols you have learnt to send energy to that person.

Chapter 5: Crystal/Pyramid And Its Treatment Methods

13.1. Introduction

Even natural stones have curing capabilities. Scientifically speaking, a crystal can store electro magnetic energy. Having a crystal ever in your pockets allows the crystal, natural friend of a human, to transmit the cosmic energy into the human body.

13.2. Cosmic Energy latent in Precious Stones

The cosmic energy can also be used along with the aid of crystals and precious stones. The results fall under three categories: The naturally found curing capabilities of crystals, coupled with the vibrations of the different colours it exhibits, quickly heal the afflictions of the person.

When cosmic energy is transmitted through crystals and precious gems, more energy is stored apart from dispelling mental depression and bodily afflictions. The powerful rays of the colours of the gems enter our body to activate the dormant energy centres and rejuvenate the whole system. Thus the twin usage of transmitting cosmic energy via gems and crystals is an experientially beneficial and healthy method of combating health disorders.

Having said this it is not mandatory to purchase costly gems. Low-cost crystals can produce the same results as the costly gems. If only costly gems can give the desired results and bring healthy trends, then the rich alone who can afford to buy the precious gems should be healthy. But this is not the case. Even the rich are often tormented by perennial health problems. Hence, money has no place in getting cured; getting cured lies in the treatment provided. Economically and naturally, cosmic energy therapy offers a healthy way to stay fit and fine.

13.3. Crystal Therapy Brings Mental Peace
Crystals are the personification of Mother Earth's equitable constructive energy. Described as a giant step towards prosperity, the continuous use of cosmic energy with crystals begets one with bliss, happiness, content and, most importantly, health for people and those around them.

Initially my experience with a quartz stone left me speechless about its potency. I placed it on my heart centre of energy and felt a big hole drilled into it. The next five minutes, I felt insects flying inside me and soon my heart drew inside to a level of absolute tranquility. This experience was too much for my intellectual belief that I ultimately understood the natural potency these stones can produce.

13.4. Crystals in Curing

After purifying the crystals under the sun for one full day, place it on the palms to charge it with the cosmic energy for 10 minutes. In this process the cosmic energy passes from your hand to the crystal, attains more potency, and reaches the target energy centres to activate them. Keeping the crystal in the palm strengthens the thumb and the tips of the fingers with cosmic energy. A crystal can also be lent to others for self-cure but it is advisable to purify it again before its next usage.

Though a crystal can be used effectively to address specific problems by placing it on that part of the body, it may also be used to transform energy from your body to another person's body with the crystal acting as a mediator between yourselves.

Crystals are endowed with seven varying colours of red, orange, yellow, green, blue, indigo, violet and white which are considered to be synonymous to the seven energy centres found in the body. The red colour is attributed to the first chakra of Mooladhara; the orange, the second colour to the second chakra and the rest to the rest of the chakras.

Transmission of cosmic energy through crystals or gems is best suited for effective results. Similarly a crystal chain of beads or a dollar shaped bead of suitable colour enhances the chances of attracting pristine energy and at the same time relieving the body of negative vibrations, thus keeping the body and soul in a well-balanced equilibrium.

13.5.   Pyramid   Therapy
Celebrated as the seventh wonder of the world,   the
Pyramid increases the emission of cosmic

energy. A pyramid made of plastic, when placed on the afflicted part, banks on the cosmic energy to the maximum and immediately relieves the pain. For instance, many Malaysian homes are designed like Pyramids; even if we sit upright with both hands rested on the laps it portrays the posture of a pyramid shape. Though this is better, the Padmaasana posture advocated in the school of Yoga is considered the best in transmitting cosmic energy.

Pyramids are rightly hailed as the Microprocessor of cosmic energy as they purify the cosmic rays. Further the pyramids can be placed in the pockets or under the pillow before going to sleep.

13.6. Crystal/Pyramid and Its Curing Techniques 13.6.1. First Level – Cleansing (in Saltwater)

Soak the crystal in salt water for 8 hours and take it out to clean it in pure water before usage. In general 7 colours are used in crystal therapy. As mentioned earlier, each colour represents each chakra or energy centre. Hence all seven crystals should be cleaned with salt water for 8 hours and then with pure water immediately. Apart from these, 7 plastic pyramids are also used but avoid cleaning these in water. Endowed with a natural cleaning instinct, salt water purifies all the negative vibrations absorbed by the crystals when under the earth. In truth, salt water is the best cleansing agent in the world.

13.6.2. Second Level – Cosmic Energy Cleanses

After placing the seven crystals and seven coloured pyramids in the left palm, we charge them with cosmic energy for five minutes to purify them of all impurities.

We can feel the heat generated on our palms by the presence of crystals and pyramids.

13.6.3. Third Level – Infusing Energy

The main aim of this crystal/pyramid therapy is the cleansing of our seven energy centres. After duly charging the pyramids/crystals with cosmic energy by placing them on the left palm, we start instilling the following thought into them by retaining the same posture of the palm.

"O Mother Cosmic Energy! Please bestow me with absolute success on this noble venture of infusing cosmic energy into the pyramid/crystals to cleanse my energy centres."

This benign thought ensures that the cosmic energy penetrates quickly into the pyramid/crystals.

13.6.4. Fourth Level – Positioning of the Chakras

Directing the healer student to lie on a bed, position each pyramid/crystal on the energy centres.

The first energy centre (chakra) is Mooladhara situated on the spine end. The attribute of this chakra is red; hence the pyramid and the crystal on top of it is positioned on this chakra.

Next comes Svadhisthanaa, the centre of water, situated 2 inches below the belly button. Orange is its attribute and, hence the orange pyramid with the orange crystal on top of it is kept in that position.

The next chakra is Manipura, just above the belly button. Position the yellow pyramid and the crystal on top of it on this place.

Fourthly, the Anagathaa, the heart centre. Colour is green and rightly so, green pyramid and the crystal are placed carefully on the heart centre.

The next chakra is throat with the blue as its colour. Position the blue pyramid and the crystal on the depth of the throat pit.

Sixth is the temple. Ajna chakra with the indigo is its attribute. Carefully place the indigo pyramid and the crystal on the temple. Beware it should not fall down.

The last and the seventh chakra is the turiya or the sahasraraa. Since the violet or white coloured crystal/pyramid cannot be positioned on a lying posture, it may be pasted on that position or kept very near to it on the bed.

Thus all the seven colours pertaining to the seven energy centres have been duly placed on the chakras.

13.6.5. Fifth Level – Relax for 10 Minutes

Now the all-important stage of infusing energy has arrived. Starting from the head down to the first chakra in Mooladhara, we can slowly wave or touch with our hand. Whenever the energy is channelised through the pyramid/crystal, the energy flow increases. Each centre is endowed with a gland and the infused cosmic energy purifies the gland associated with each centre and makes it produce the hormones properly. Even if certain blockages are present in some centres, it is removed by the introduction of these powerful energy waves, just like snow melts in the presence of sun's rays.

Our body gets light and the surprising fact is the purification of all the seven energy centres and the equilibrium created. Energising for 10 minutes ensures the required 6 inches diameter of aura of each energy centre with varying colours.

13.6.6. Sixth Level – Thanks giving

After invoking the thanksgiving gesture to the Almighty for his grace in the success of the therapy, slowly displace the pyramids/crystals from their positions.

13.7. The Four Ways in which this Therapy works

1. The crystal's curing capabilities.
2. The colour of the rays.
3. The potency of the pyramids.
4. The power of cosmic energy.

These four attributes work together to do wonders and maintain equilibrium. Constant practice brings mastery and a separate set of pyramids/crystals is advised for curing outside patients. Though the same pyramid/crystal may be applied for treating others, enough care has to be adopted such as purifying them properly before use, in saltwater, wiping them with a clean cloth and recharging with cosmic energy. A word of warning: Since the crystals have high degree of absorbing capabilities, a un-cleaned crystal used on one patient stands the risk of communicating the affliction to another person, as the crystals retain the vibrations of the patient it was used last on.

13.8. Laser Energy

Apart from serving as a tool of cure of diseases, the crystals act as energy carriers. The laser energy therapy, as it is known, operates when placed on the afflicted part by emitting a powerful energy wave and relieves it of pain.

13.9. Power of the Pyramid

As already mentioned, the time-tested pyramid technique is the seventh wonder of the world. The most amazing factor is how the Egyptians could conceive such an astounding invention during those times when science and technological breakthroughs were unheard of. Though everyone agrees rightly with the claim that these pyramids were used to preserve the dead bodies of the kings (Pharos), it is still a puzzle even to the historians why the ancient Egyptians chose to design them in the pyramid shape and built them with the use of Alabaster stones. It is a bewildering fact that these pyramids have stood the test of time and never ever showed signs of wear and tear even when faced with umpteen earthquakes, heavy rain, scorching heat over the centuries. Some unseen power is sure to lie behind this massive structure that surpasses human intelligence. This secret needs to be unveiled by the scientists. Does science have any answer to this?

13.10. Usage of Pyramids

It is a scientifically proven fact that items kept inside this pyramid structure remain fresh for many days. The second experiment proved even more effective with a blade becoming sharper with no signs of rust, when kept in a pyramid. Even a rusted blade retained its sharpness for 6 days inside the pyramid. So pyramid's greatness lies in the energy it releases. Let us now examine how these structures called pyramids can be effectively used to enhance our lives. A pyramid's height, length, breadth and its dimension are all important. It is simple to make these pyramids in any material of your choice, be it plastic, metal, crystal, wood or paper. What matters is the measurement. Any size is sure to increase the nutrient content of the preserved food and distil the water's impurities and clean it for usage.

A pyramid's size: Height = 1 foot; Breadth = 1.5708 foot; side slope = 1.4945 foot.

13.11. To Perform Meditation

A meditation performed inside a pyramid-shaped room ensures a tranquil and effective state of mind. It purifies the air inside it and creates an ambience in the person's mind. This does not mean that we perform meditation only inside pyramids; the same atmosphere can be effectively created where you stay.

Tie the pyramid-shaped object, just above the head and sit for meditation. Irrespective of the size of the pyramid, it brings concentration and relieves the pain from the afflicted part if placed on that. Pyramid soothes the mind and effects good sleep. Further tying 4 to 5 pyramids on the ceiling of the bedroom filters the negative vibrations and produces a conducive environment for a refreshing sleep. Even water preserved inside a pyramid can be used to nurture plants and flowers. Pyramids, when placed in bathrooms, act as a room refresher and activate the positive vibrations.

13.12. Pyramids for Life's Aim

When pyramids are used to transmit cosmic energy, it doubles the impact on us. Pyramids placed in purses and money bags ensure safety of the money in transit. Further the aim of life is best achieved when cosmic energy therapy via the pyramid is practised to maximise the effects. When the desired aim is written in a paper and kept between two pyramids to infuse cosmic energy, the written aim assumes life and materialises. This sums up the scintillating effect of the pyramids, the Egyptians' outstanding contribution to this world.

13.13. Pyramids – Protective Force

Pyramids act as protective force in all places and at all times. Be it in a public transport, train or during air travel, the pyramid protection ensures a safe journey for you and your belongings. Houses are burglar-proofed and protected against negative forces when guarded by a pyramid. This can also be effectively used to guard children and old people.

Chapter 6: The Second Chakra

Once your first chakra is open, you will have an easier time opening the rest of your chakras. Remember that once you decide to go on this journey of opening your chakras, you can never turn back. The opening of an individual's chakras is an intense and personal journey that allows anyone to become in touch with their inner, real selves. This chapter will introduce you to the second chakra.

Water Chakra

The second chakra is also known as the water chakra or the sacral chakra. It deals mainly with pleasure, and is blocked by the emotion of guilt. The second chakra point is located behind and just below the navel.

The water chakra is mainly associated with an individual's sexuality. It also governs creativity and a sense of childlike wonder. Now, while these two concepts may seem to clash, you must understand that creativity and childlike wonder is often thought to be fully expressed through a person's deeper understanding about his or her sexuality. This maturation while retaining the innocence of a child is often blocked by taboos and norms that prohibit self-expression through the experience of pleasure and desire.

However, this is not to say that the second chakra is empowered or recharged by mindless sexual acts and engagement in destructive relationships. Instead, the second chakra is empowered through sexual and pleasurable acts that stem from a profound relationship that is not afraid to reach past the boundaries imposed by the world and its people. It is empowered by a love that surpasses the neediness, the selfishness and jealousy that most immature relationships experience. It is empowered by a love that is complete in and of itself, instead of dependent on another individual's attentions.

Opening the water chakra

As you must have already guessed, the water chakra is positively affected by staying in water, drinking water. To open the water chakra you can follow these simple steps:

Step 1: Find a calm, quiet place where you can be alone and focus on the task ahead of you. The place you choose should have free access to water. Most people open their water chakras in the privacy of their bathrooms, or in the freedom of a swimming pool or beach. Choose a place where you won't hesitate to be yourself, where you won't be awkward or too conscious about what you are doing.

Choose a place where you can be one with the water.

Step 2: Once you find a quiet place, sit or stand comfortably. Breathe slowly and deeply, releasing your doubts, fears and inhibitions. Clear your mind.

Step 3: Let the water run or shower you with its coolness. If you are in a pool or the beach, find a way to make the water touch you or submerge you.

Step 4: Think about the things you have done, the people and the places that have helped you experience pleasure, no matter how simple or complicated. Picture them in your mind. Keep breathing slowly and deeply.

Step 5: Now think about the guilt that plagues you. What things, people or events have made you feel guilty? What choices and decisions have contributed to your guilt?

Step 6: Once you have both the things that have made you feel pleasure and guilt, begin to release them one by one. Let them flow with the water. Let the water wash away your guilt, and rejuvenate your strength. Imagine the second chakra point opening, and glowing as you allow the water to cleanse and strengthen it.

Step 7: Inhale and exhale. Keep the cleansed, empowered feeling that the water has shared with you. Finish opening your chakra by clearing your mind once more, and then slowly opening your eyes to face the realities of the world.

The water chakra is also recharged by contact with the color orange, and by eating melons, walnuts, passion fruits and almonds. Remember that the water chakra teaches forgiveness and acceptance. Only by accepting that blame and guilt are part of everyday life will you be able to understand why you must never be clouded by them.

Chapter 7: The Difference Between Reiki And Angelic Reiki

Synopsis

There are a lot of deviations between the Reiki systems that are taught in the world and Angelic Reiki.

It's now typically accepted that the system of healing called Reiki is the original system of healing that was used in Atlantis. It's widely accepted that the civilization of Atlantis was elevated in consciousness in regards to contacting Divine Wisdom than our society nowadays.

They utilized vibrational symbols to reach divine powers which when used in a closed system, like the body, would cause balance and alignment. This is the way healing arrives.

The Differences

The healing system of the Atlantian's was rediscovered by Dr Usui in the 1880s, due to humans now being on the opposite of the 26,000 year cycle of our solar system, where Atlantis was demolished.

The system of healing that Dr Usui rediscovered has been stringently preserved through the lineage of the purity of transmission of the symbols that Dr Usui used.

The spiritual percept of humanity in the 1880s embraced the fact that we were part of a system called the Solar System. What this means is that intellectual/spiritual human race at that time could only comprehend themselves to be part of the Solar System. The symbols that Dr Usui used were given out to utilize with the vibration of humans at that time, which was solar consciousness.

Since the 1880s, humanity has amplified in consciousness at a quickened rate. After World War 2, a leap in consciousness let humans expand consciousness to adopt the fact that we're one solar system in a galaxy of a lot of solar systems. This might be termed galactic consciousness. All of the Reiki schemes which have developed since this time have built on the traditional Reiki symbols, and given those symbols equate with the heart chakra.

Since the Harmonic Convergence of 1987, a different leap in consciousness resulted which has let the Reiki symbols be given at higher vibrations than heart chakra.

Once Angelic Reiki was first conducted in 2003, the attunements to the symbols were happening at the throat chakra vibration. Recently, for the first time since Atlantian times the healing symbols of Atlantis have the chance of being used at the full 7 levels of form and Divine Form.

In Angelic Reiki all of the symbols used, are used through the complete 7 levels of form and Divine form.

From time immemorial, with all of the mystery school traditions, activations in consciousness have been presented by the Master to the pupil through initiation.

Before initiations were presented the pupil had to prove, frequently through physical trial, their worthiness to get the initiation. This practice has been fairly diluted by the New-Age Movement.

An initiation is an energetic attunement of the Masters consciousness impressed up on the consciousness of the pupil. It's a merging; an over lighting of one consciousness by another, in order to elevate the vibration and awareness of that consciousness into the beaming light of the Master.

A few of the attunements given nowadays through the Reiki system are not of the highest. The pupil receiving such an initiation may open themselves to be imprinted by a consciousness that is still going through egoic issues, emotional drama and personality bonds.

The Angelic Reiki system has always stood for a system of healing, that through the utilization of symbols which channel Divine Archetypal Energies, will attune the 7 bodies of man to their original divine vibration.

So that these symbols are channeled to pupils in their purity, they're not given as an initiation by the teacher. That teacher opens up a space, a vortex of power, whereby the Angelic Kingdom evidences their energy around each pupil and anchors the symbols into the suitable chakras.

The symbols are thereby given at divine vibration, and as such, impact the consciousness of each pupil from the minute they're given.

In this system of rules there are the traditional initiations, 1 through 4. As well, there are 2 other initiations which are strictly angelic.

The angelic kingdom was produced as part of an earlier evolution of this universe. There is, consequently, a vast difference between the vibration of an Angel and the vibration of an incarnated human.

This being accepted, the Archangel Metatron took a firm stand that an initiation into the angelic vibration be an inbuilt part of this system.

It's my understanding that through these initiations the atomic spin of each molecule in the human body of the pupil getting this attunement is sped up. This helps the energy of the pupil to more perfectly meld with the energy of the angels which are their constant companions following this initiation.

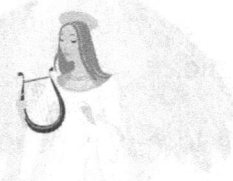

Chapter 8: Reiki Tips For Beginners

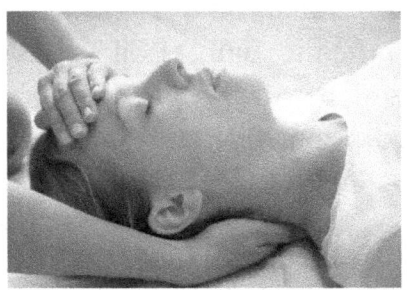

Spiritual healing is very important if you want to live a balanced life filled with joy and harmony. A balanced life refers to being abundant and content in all aspects such as career, wealth, health, relationships and personal fulfillment.

What people do not usually realize is sometimes even when problems seem to have no relationship with one another, on a deeper level they do. For example, if you are unhappy with your job, if your health is failing or are having problems with your relationships, although they may seem to be caused by different reasons, they are actually an indication of a deeper and more significant pain. Reiki is a natural method which you can perform so you can tap into your energy and heal all aspects of your life.

Those who perform Reiki testify to how well it can treat illnesses, relieve pain, reduce stress, curb cravings, promote calm and increase energy. The good thing about Reiki is you can perform it on yourself, once a Reiki master has taught you. One of the best tips of Reiki self-healing is for you to take your time in performing the different exercises. Do them slowly and make sure that you are relaxed and calm. While performing the exercises, it would help if you visualize the energy flowing through your body, especially into the areas where you need improvement.

Doing so will help you relax more and make you more aware of your body.

Another useful tip is to make sure that you choose the right time and suitable place to perform Reiki. Consistency is key to reap the benefits, so make an effort to set aside at least a few minutes of your time every day. An hour every day is ideal but if you are too busy, 15 minutes will do. If you have been feeling sluggish and want to increase your energy levels, it is best to perform Reiki in the morning. Doing so will energize and invigorate you. If you feel super stressed out after a long day at work, Reiki can help you unwind once you get home. Find a place where you cannot be distracted or disturbed for a certain period time. You should spend your session focusing solely on your body and the techniques you are performing. Remember, a quiet space and comfortable position are essential.

For Reiki to be effective, you need to be able to meditate with no distractions. Therefore, before proceeding with your session, take some time to clear your mind and let go of negative thoughts. Focus on your breathing and take deep breaths. Inhale through your nose and then slowly exhale through your nose as well.

Learn the different hand positions, as they are vital in focusing your attention on the different parts of your body. One of Reiki's goals is to unblock the flow of energy in chakras or centers where tension, pressure and stress are intensely felt, but feel free to redirect your efforts on body parts that might be needing attention.

Unlike massages, Reiki only requires a light touch on the chakras. Each touch should be light, relaxed and effortless. The good thing about Reiki is that you will already see and feel the difference after one session. However, to make the most out of the benefits of Reiki, it is recommended to take some time every day to perform the different exercises. When you are able to reduce and let go of the stress your body experiences every day, it will naturally improve its ability to resist diseases and illnesses. Do not be discouraged if you miss one or two sessions. If you missed, just simply pick up where you left off. A few minutes every day will help you maintain the benefits of Reiki.

While Reiki can be used as a self-healing tool, it also works very well as a complementary method instead of treating it as a substitute for conventional medicine and treatments. Reiki has become extremely useful and has been proven to improve the lives and health of people diagnosed with various medical conditions by relieving the pain and reducing the symptoms. However, it is not recommended that you abandon or not undergo treatments and take prescription medications.

Chapter 9: Health Benefits Of Reiki

Reiki has shown in tremendous ways that it helps in putting people's health in top shape. Although a simple process, it usually produces profound and remarkable results. Clients, far and wide, attested that Reiki sessions can help them to get by avalanches of health quagmires which include cases of infertility, deep-seated anxiety, and chronic depression, among others. The effect and results as seen from clients that have experienced Reiki treatment show that its benefit in the human life is in many folds: It affects all its compartments from physical to mental, emotional and even spiritual.

Benefits

By now you definitely know already that Reiki's energy is non-invasive, and it is absolutely effective—promoting overall body's well-being and enhancing the inherent ability of the human body to self-heal. Balances and perfect congruence are restored at all levels and instead of just masking or relieving symptoms, it works directly on the health condition.

You are on your way to an assured and pacific state if you have an unvarying Reiki treatment—and you can as well be sure that a calmer and less-tensed being is the eventuality. Reiki treatments promote a natural equilibrium and perfect alignment between the body, mind, and soul, dissolves energy blockages in the body, and leave you a being primed to cope better with the rigors of mental imbalances and clarity.

With Reiki, you are guaranteed to win the fight against tension and stress as it provides for you a window through which you will be versed with the ongoing in your total being because the session gets you into alignment with the universe energy.

Nothing helps your body in its quest to resist diseases and all manner of ills through self-cleansing from toxins and immune-defense like the touch of Reiki treatments.

Perhaps it comes to a point in time where you really need to raise tour game to a level where you maintain a clear-minded and laser-focused concentration as you feel grounded. Try Reiki because it will really help you stayed focused in the present moment—far beyond dwindling between that which had been or that which is yet to be. Even when outcomes do not appear as you have planned, you would still have gained the ability to accept and deal with the way things are unfolding.

There is no best way to go if you want to improve your sleep as a Reiki session as the number one outcome from such an astonishing experience is relaxation. Our complete being heals better when we are very relaxed, our minds become laced with clarity and purpose and there is a new wave of genuineness that permeates our relationship with other humans.

Improvement in your mood automatically decreases chances of anxiety and worry and that is what Reiki does to you. By the time you have positive energy flowing within you—something that increases your positive vibrations and keeps you in alignment, your spirit and level of excitement increases exponentially as a result.

With Reiki, the body is helped to relatively combat and reduce inflammation levels and improve the conditions precipitated in the body by infection. Those who have had surgeries and others suffering from the risk of different kinds of infections are mostly the beneficiaries.

Reiki is said to be effective when it comes to treating issues that border on joints—both in range of motion and health—in the human body. Under regular Reiki treatments, the pain that comes from a migraine and arthritis can be dealt with superbly.

Heard of metabolic syndrome? It means a collection of diseases verily, as research has proven, linked to serious conditions like diabetes, heart disease, among others. Reiki helps reduce its risk and deal with any side conditions effectively.

What a great self-care tool Reiki is. What this means is that, through wielding the force imbued in Reiki, you have mastered how to be one with the universe and utilize its healing energy for good.

Your blood gets happy under a Reiki session. According to a study, those who had a Reiki session timeout, compared to those who were just unperturbed, were found to have an increased volume of white blood cells. Do you really know what that means for your health? It means Reiki treatments natural increases the body's natural immune ability to fend off illness, wade off dangerous infections, and self-heal.

Cancer, like HIV Aids, comes with a barrage of other ills, anxieties, pain, depression, among others and these are conditions powerful Reiki sessions are renowned for taking away.

For those who are just coming out of surgery or recovering from a long-term illness, Reiki is a bargain. It helps fight off side effects (vomiting, nausea) of medicinal treatments as recorded especially in patients just out of chemotherapy.

If you ever suffer a burn or a scar, then Reiki is the way out as it helps to accelerate tissues regeneration, making the spots as though it was never stressed or peeled away. Reiki's ability to enhance tissue regeneration makes is connected to its ability to revitalize the body cells in slowing down the aging process.

According to testimonials from pregnant women and mothers, Reiki served them well. It was very helpful in reducing complications during childbirth and pregnancy.

With Reiki, you gain a great advantage in that your human mind finds natural alignment with higher universal forces. A deeper gift of connection with your Higher Self and a new wave of spiritual enlightenment/growth is a reward for using Reiki.

Chapter 10: Maintaining The Vibration Of A Healer In The Face Of Daily Life

By Tracy Morrow

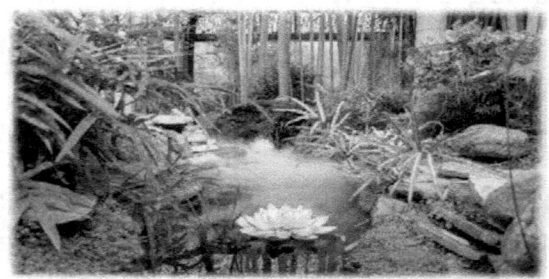

As we train to become Reiki practitioners, we learn how to begin living the Principles, become attuned to the utterly beautiful and subtle energies that we had been previously blocked from, and learn to share the energy with others. This is done as a journey which at first calls us to leave our normal life behind while we study and practice. Along this new path our identity expands to include our newfound skills and way of life. Yet, merging this new identity into the rest of our life can seem quite challenging. In fact, it is common for most practitioners to wonder how to better maintain the vibration of a Healer in the face of daily life.

While even the most dedicated practitioner will spend time in reflection of the Reiki Principles every morning, clear their energy and invite Reiki into their day, the day seems to quickly take over. An accumulation of events call out for our attention and at some point we realize we have resorted to operating from lower energy realms. We may find ourselves acting out in anger, succumbing to stress symptoms or otherwise acting and feeling very "un-healer like". We may even begin to doubt if we even have an ability to truly be a healer or not. Fortunately, most of what we struggle with is our own minds. Let's look at how to overcome that.

Awareness and acceptance are two of the most integral qualities to develop as a Reiki practitioner. Awareness that you are an emotional creature and will continue to experience darker emotions such as anger, resentment, stress and so forth allows the space to accept those feelings with equanimity. This acceptance is paramount as all emotions are deserving of our compassion. Where we may stumble is in reflecting on the Reiki principles. These principles admonish you to not anger or worry. This does not mean to refuse to allow the emotions of anger and concern. Instead, it means to refrain from becoming or acting out in those emotions.

When you embrace darker emotions, you are able to hear the messages they offer. Anger for instance, is a great message that says that a boundary needs to be set. That boundary can be set in love and using the highest energy of a healer.

You can refrain from becoming the emotion of anger, while still accepting it is a part of you. This goes the same for any other emotion that you might think is "un-healer" like. Find the message in the emotion, treat it with Reiki and choose the healthiest response, even if that response is to accept that there is nothing to do other than cradle the emotion with compassion until it subsides.

As you develop awareness and acceptance of what inhibits you from maintaining a higher vibration in the face of daily life, surrendering becomes an integral activity. Specifically, surrendering the resistance of what is. When you capitulate to the present moment, exactly how it presents itself, and aside from expectations or how you might like to control it, you will find great peace. Surrendering in this way grants the power to respond to the moment from a higher vibration, instead of reacting out of old, and perhaps dysfunctional, habits.

Awareness, acceptance, and surrender will allow you to excel in maintaining the vibration of a Healer in the face of daily life. Therefore, practicing these qualities takes on a profound importance. Pursuing activities such as remaining diligent with the Reiki principles, taking time for meditation, yoga and other mindfulness exercises will help you strengthen these qualities. As you gently guide yourself daily within these practices, they will begin to naturally spill over into the rest of your life. Before you realize it, you will be maintaining high vibrations no matter what the moments of your day present to you.

Reiki Ball for Healing

By Haripriya Suraj

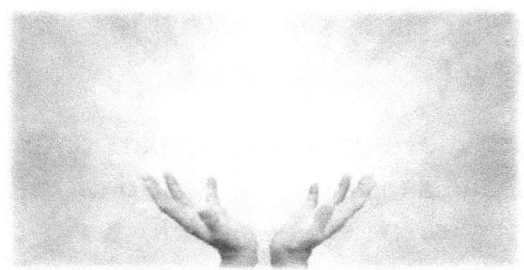

A Reiki ball, also known as an energy ball, is a very useful healing tool. In simple terms, a Reiki ball can be described as a chunk of Reiki that is brought together in the form of a ball. It comes in handy in a variety of situations. It is a tool that can keep Reiki flowing to people or situations. There is no limit to how creative one can get while working with Reiki balls!

How to Make a Reiki Ball

For those hearing this for the first time, here's how you make a ball of Reiki.

Rub your palms for a few seconds until you experience sensations of warmth.

Curve your palms slightly so it resembles a flower bud.

Begin to move your palms apart until you feel strong sensations of heat or a kind of magnetic force between them.

Move your palms up and down in circular motion, like you would if you were carving a ball. Feel or visualise a ball of energy between them.

If you are attuned to symbols, infuse the ball with the symbols of your choice. Visualise the symbols in the ball and it will be done.

Don't worry if you can't feel much initially. As you practise, you will be able to sense the ball in your hands.

Uses of a Reiki Ball

The following ideas serve as a reference to help you get started. With practice, you will find that the possibilities for healing with Reiki balls are virtually endless.

Affirmations

If you work with affirmations for healing, place a Reiki ball over the affirmation or on the page that has your writing.

Reiki Box

Whenever you work with your Reiki box, place a ball of Reiki in it. This will keep your intentions continuously charged with Reiki. If your Reiki box is in your phone, push the ball into the Reiki Box App.

Physical Healing

When there is a need for physical healing, push a ball of Reiki into the affected body part. In the case of internal organs, push the ball into the body, just over the location of the organ. Intend that the ball goes into the affected organ and heals it.

Pain Relief

If pain relief is needed, program the Reiki ball with the intention that it heals pain. Then push it into the body part or organ that needs relief from pain.

Spread Love

If you wish to send your love to someone, program a Reiki ball with the intention of sending love and toss it into the air. Pink being the colour of love, you can also visualise pink light inside the ball. Intend that the ball goes to the person and makes him or her feel loved. The other person may not consciously realise what happened. They may just experience feelings of love and warmth when the ball reaches them. This practice can bring in more love and harmony to all relationships.

Romantic Love

Program a ball with the intention of sending romantic love to your partner or spouse. Throw in some pink light as well. Toss the ball into the air. Intend that the ball reaches your beloved and conveys your unconditional love and acceptance to your partner.

Comfort

Whenever you are in emotional pain, program a Reiki ball with the mental-emotional symbol and Master Symbol (if you've done third degree). Throw in some pink light and push it into your heart chakra. You can also push it into other parts of your body as you feel guided to. Intend that it brings you comfort and peace. Let go and witness the spontaneous healing that occurs.

Protection

Program a Reiki ball with the Power Symbol and Master Symbol (if you've done third degree). Intend that it stays with any object, place or person that needs protection. Place it over your house, over babies and children and over your belongings. You could send it along with a loved one who is travelling. Place it over your vehicle whenever you travel. Place it over food and water.

Plants and Animals

Place balls of Reiki over plants in your garden. Push them into trees. Intend that the energy helps your plants stay healthy and nurtures your garden. Place it over a pet or other animal that is unwell or needs protection.

Finding Misplaced Objects

If you've misplaced something, make a ball of Reiki and request it to go in search of the missing object. Toss it into the air and visualise it going away in search of the misplaced object. Thereafter, pay attention to your intuition. You may receive clues as to where the object is or you may see the location of the object in your mind's eye. Trust the impressions you receive and look for the object as guided to. It can also happen that you are physically directed to the place that has the misplaced object.

Cleansing

Program a ball of Reiki with the power symbol. Toss it into rooms and other spaces that have accumulated negative energies. To thoroughly cleanse a room, place a ball of Reiki in each corner of the room. Push a ball of Reiki into the walls, the floor, the ceiling, windows, doors, wardrobes etc.

Now it's time for you to get creative and experiment with Reiki Balls! Let your imagination run wild. Have fun!

Chapter 11: Karma/Blockages

What is Karma?

How our thoughts, actions and words determine our present Karma?

How does Karma work?

What are different types of Karma?

What is Karma?

Karma = Cause and Effect.

Karma is action that is driven by a person's intention.

Literally translated, the word Karma means "**action**". It comes from the Sanskrit root '**kr**,' which means "**to act**". The Karma includes movement of our body and thoughts. According to Buddhist tradition, Karma refers to action that is driven by a person's intention.

"For every action there is an equal or opposite reaction."

The 3 major things we have to keep in check:

Mind – Thoughts

Feelings – Actions

Intention – Words

Karma is the result of our thoughts, actions and words.

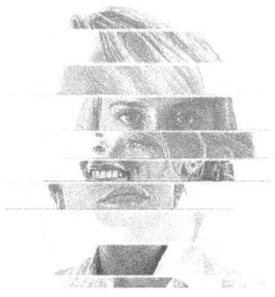

How our thoughts, actions and words determine our present Karma?

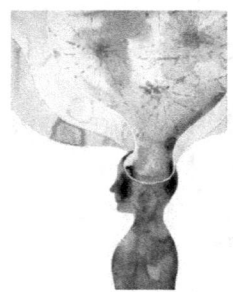

"Our thoughts and feelings shape the world within us [physical body], our words and actions shape the world around us [Magnetic field/Aura]".

Thought is a process of thinking. The thoughts we think either positive or negative will be determined by our mindset. Mind is mesmerizing; It controls the way we view our self, (the ego), and everything around us. The mind never rests; it continuously process, recognize, and evaluates the information even when we are asleep.

Our thoughts determine our basic nature. Positive thoughts about oneself or others lead to positive way of living, whereas negative thoughts create bad Karma. Every thought we think creates our future. The movement we realize that things don't have to be in a certain way, we get rid of expectations, self-doubt, criticism and shame, so why to indulge in a negative thought? Release the negative thought, let go and feel free.

Action here refers to our behavior or the way we physically react to any situation. Our actions easily define our character. Never let circumstances determine your actions. Cultivate conscious action, so that you will never add up bad Karma because of your actions. Any action performed according to dharma without any personal gain, likes or dislikes is called Karma-yoga. No matter whatever we learn, know or say it is useless; until we put it into the right action.

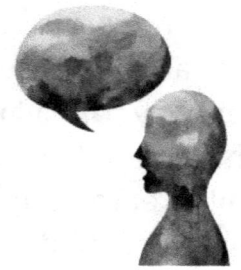

Example: Knowledge, understanding, commitment, love, affection, care remain words and mean nothing if your actions are opposite to it. So put your knowledge, patience, affection, care and love into action and see how natural healing works.

Words or what we talk should be positive, never carry feeling of resentment and hurt others. Before you react or say something, think how you'd feel if the same was said to you. Words carry power, power to heal and feel good. Hurting a good person with your words creates a bad Karma whereas keeping quite towards myth also. Kind words cost nothing.

When we start to think, act and speak according to dharma. We start to clear our Karma instead of accumulating a little more.

How does Karma work?

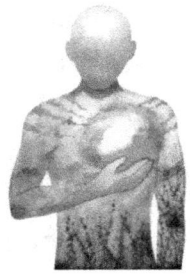

Karma can effect mentally, physically or can even cause emotional pain. Karma can be positive or negative, it reflects from our sub-conscious mind. Karma is not a punishment, it is an invisible power that teaches and helps us to understand where we went wrong. The purpose of Karma is to help us to change for good.

Karma is an unbreakable rule of the cosmos. We are solely responsible for our actions, whether good or bad, all thoughts and actions are powerful and they carry energy any action either positive/negative have consequences.

Sometimes Karma reflects immediately and in other cases it might be delayed but no matter how long it takes, there will always be an effect. So, if you keep doing good things with the best of intentions, later you will also experience the best of what life has to offer.

Karma is not always negative, there are positive Karma's too based on ones actions and mindset, they reach out us in the journey of life as unexpected blessings.

Types of Karma

Yogically, there are 3 types of Karma. The Karma of the past, present and future are called as Sanchita, Prabdha and Agami Karma.

Sanchita Karma [List of unresolved past actions waiting for final results]

Sanchita Karma is storehouse of all our good and bad deeds.

In simple terms it is accumulated Karma of our previous lifetimes. All good or bad deeds from past lives flows through next lives.

Prabdha Karma [Present actions]

Prabdha has no waiting, the result is now. It is the part of sanchita Karma, a collection of past Karmas, which has to be experienced through the present body.

Prabdha Karma will be based on our thoughts and actions at the present.

Agami Karma [Future actions]

When we attempt to resolve a past Karma, we unavoidably create new Karmas through our thoughts and actions, we may or may not be able to resolve it in our present life.

This left out or unresolved Karma will be stored and will be resolved in a future life.

Agami Karma is also called as future Karma.

Karma is perfect, unbreakable universal law. We can't stop it, but we can change its direction by, dropping hatred, guilt and grudge, learning from past mistakes or problems we have faced and by accepting positive changes, we can change our present situation.

The only way to erase bad Karma is by regretting, learning from it and by practising kindness and love. There is no other way.

Chapter 12: Treating Others With Reiki

In this book, we will look at the practice of treating others with Reiki through the aura or energy field. Many practitioners believe that treating through the aura is most effective (more effective than physical touch) as Reiki will enter the aura first and easily move through the energy field to the place it is most needed. If you recall from earlier chapters, illness can derive from disharmony or blockage in the aura (or due to thoughts and emotions), so treating the aura can treat illnesses at their root or before they take hold in the physical body.

You may even find that you prefer to conduct your self-treatments through the aura rather than with physical touch. Use your intuition to guide you.

The following steps can be used to guide you in treating others with Reiki. Reiki can be used on both people and animals.

Set your intention to heal and allow the Reiki to flow through you. To do so, place your hands together in the prayer position in front of your chest and concentrate on the flow of Reiki.

Set intentions and expectations for the treatment with the other person. Make sure they are comfortable and know what to expect during the treatment. Before beginning the treatment have the client close their eyes and meditate on accepting healing energies.

Do not bring pre-conceived notions. The Reiki will go where it is needed, you are the conduit for the healing, not the director. Remember, Reiki will not diminish your ki, or energy, instead it will also heal and cleanse you as you use it.

In many states, individuals who are not licensed healthcare practitioners may not touch the physical body of another during treatment. This is another reason why aura treatments may be preferred.

Refer to the images in Chapter 4 on self-treatment as a guide for hand placement in treating others. Remember, there are many different hand placements used in Reiki, these positions are a starting point. Follow the positions, then use your intuition to add or remove as the Reiki guides you.

Hand Position 1

Place your hands, palms down, fingers together, one to four inches above the face.

Hand Position 2

Place your hands one to four inches over from the ears.

Hand Position 3

Place your hands one to four inches above the collar bone.

Hand Position 4

Place your hands one to four inches above the crown of the head.

Hand Position 5

Place your right hand one to four inches above the neck and your left hand one to four inches above the heart.

Hand Position 6

Place your hands one to four inches above the rib cage.

Hand Position 7

Place your hands one to four inches above the solar plexus.

Hand Position 8

Place your hands one to four inches above the stomach.

Hand Position 9

Place your hands one to four inches above the lower abdomen and pubic bones.

Hand Position 10

Place your hands one to four inches above the knees.

Hand Position 11

Place your hands one to four inches above the soles of the feet.

Hand Position 12

Place your right hand one to four inches above the crown of the head and your left hand one to four inches above the solar plexus.

Other Positions

Again, if desired, you may treat the shoulders, middle back, lower back, and sacrum.

End the session with Reiki one to four inches above the feet for grounding.

Aura Cleansing

Clear the person's energy field by sweeping away any stagnant energies that were unblocked during the session. To do so, comb your fingers down their aura (remaining one to four inches above their body) from the crown of the head to the feet, using a sweeping motion with your hands.

When you have finished, let the person rest quietly for a few moments before getting up.

Wash your hands at the end of the session to clear away any remaining unwanted energies.

In the next chapter, we will look at affirmations and mantras for specific diseases and problems. The affirmations can be used during Reiki sessions to help the subconscious accept Reiki healing energy.

Key Take Away

Treating others with Reiki can be a gentle complimentary therapy to traditional healing. In the beginning, treat all positions. As you grow in your practice, us Reiji-Ho to intuitively treat other positions with Reiki.

A great benefit of Reiki is that Reiki guides the treatment and flows where it is needed, your only task is to get out of the way and let Reiki do its job. Also, Reiki does not use your energy or drain your energy during healing – it flows through you from the universal source – and even heals you as you channel Reiki to another.

Chapter 13: Exercises For Specific Areas Of The Body

Let's take a look at some beginner exercises to target specific areas so that you have something to work with. The more you exercise and take your time to learn the exercises correctly, the better the chances of you gleaning benefit from them. Remember, it is not a marathon and you don't get prizes for finishing quickly. The exercises take discipline and that can sometimes mean that slowness of approach is wiser.

Abs, Core and Flat Tummy

I want to introduce you to an exercise that is really useful for men and women. For men, it will help to keep the pelvic floor working as it should and for women, it will help to firm up your tummy area and help digestive problems as well. The side shoot from many yoga exercises is that they have multiple benefits. You may think that you are just exercising one part of the body, when in fact you are helping others at the same time. If your problem is between your waist and your knees, this is the exercise for you. It will help to tighten the abs. It will help to flatten the stomach but above all, it will help to strengthen those muscles that may have become lapse — either after life events such as pregnancy — or for men — when problems occur such as prostate or inability to urinate smoothly.

Let's get into position ready for this exercise, which is a lying down position. When you are lying down, don't get lazy about how your feet are placed. Imagine that you are standing up and place your feet so that they are straight and your ankle is at a right angle to the floor. This helps to strengthen your leg muscles. Now, point your toes and stretch them toward your body. This is a great way of opening up the chakras so that the energy can flow through your body as you exercise. Breathe in and breathe out and allow your body to feel really relaxed. Breathing is not just used for movement. It is also used to calm the moments between exercises.

Keeping one leg completely straight, pull the other up to your chest and put your hands around it to pull it into your chest. Then, while still holding onto your knee push it as if you want to push it away from your body but hold it firmly. What you want to feel is that wonderful resistance because this is helping focus the exercise on a specific area and that is the thigh area. Now do the same with the other side.

For the next part of this exercise sequence, be aware that your shoulders need to be firm against the mat. Your legs should be straight and your arms down by your sides with your palms spread out touching the mat. Move your feet so that they are flat against the carpet and then lift your whole body so that your back is resting on your shoulders, arms and your feet, but is lifted from the carpet. Remember, breathe in and lift, breathe out and hold the position, breathe in and settle your back onto the carpet, breath out and relax.

This time, instead of your feet being flat on the carpet, put them so that you are resting on the toes and your foot is stretched out and against lift your whole body and keep it as aligned as possible, taking the weight on your toes and your shoulders. This is great for the pelvic floor and also for getting all those muscles you haven't used that much in your lower abdomen into trim. This will help with all kinds of problems, such as digestive problems, constipation, etc. and is very beneficial to your lower back region.

Rocking your body

This is the next progression on this exercise. Lift your legs and lift them so that they are at a right angle to your body. In other words, they should be straight upward. Stretch the legs and move them toward your head and then back to their central position. No move them toward the rug away from your head. Swing them like this for a while, remembering to breathe with each movement. This rocking motion is stretching the muscles and helping your legs to feel great. Move alternate legs separately as well, because this will make your thighs feel good. As you rock both legs, make the rock more pronounced and rock yourself back up into a seated position.

These exercises are great for beginners and do not ask for much expertise.

However, exercise with caution and make sure that you do not push yourself further than you are comfortable with. Your body shouldn't hurt. You need to practice over and over again, making sure that a breath accompanies each movement. Breathe – move – Breathe. It's vital that you get that rhythm right from the beginning as the exercises that yoga instructors give get more and more complex and this breathing helps you to achieve them without too much difficulty.

At the end of the exercise, place your hands by your sides and relax. Breathe in and out.

Chapter 14: Living With An Attitude Of Gratitude

Usui's third precept is "Just for today be thankful".

Are you a thankful person?

Are you full of gratitude or do you regularly complain about your lot?

When Usui formulated this principle I believe he was asking us to do more than just say "thank you". He was asking for us to develop an attitude of gratitude.

It seems that in our society we always want to have more – a bigger house, a better car, more money, or more stuff. We say things like, "I need a new car" or "I need a new top". We are getting our needs and our wants mixed up!

We actually forget what we do have because we are constantly focusing on what we don't have. I believe Usui was asking us to focus on the blessings we have in our lives and to become grateful.

Need or want?

So how do we do this and how do we differentiate our needs from our wants?

Psychologist, Abraham Maslow, (1908-70) came up with a hierarchy of needs which I think is a useful illustration of this concept. Basing our needs on a triangle he came up with 5 groups of needs.

Starting at the base, the widest part of the triangle we have our major needs – the big things we need to actually survive – food, drink, sleep and the need to procreate. These are number 1.

Secondly then once our basic physiological needs have been met we can move to our need for safety – the need for a safe place to live, enough money to live on and psychological security.

Once those foundations are in place then we can move up the pyramid to the third set of needs – the need for love and belonging – our need for affection, intimacy and roots in our family or society.

Group four covers our need for esteem – Maslow argued that this need would only come into place once the first three sets of needs were met.

This is our need to believe in ourselves, in our competency, our self-respect and having respect for others. It may be, therefore, that if you suffer from an inability to respect yourself or to believe in yourself that your base needs are not being met.

It is only once all these needs have been met that we can move up to group 5 at the top of the pyramid – Maslow called this the need for self-actualisation – in other words, the ability to become what we are capable of becoming.

It is at this point that we feel safe and confident enough to explore more and investigate philosophical concepts and spirituality.

It is an interesting concept and one which I feel has quite a lot of merit.

If we do not meet our basic needs, then how can we try and develop ourselves spiritually or personally?

Perhaps it is time we all looked at our needs from this perspective and then we can easily identify whether our wants and our needs are the same thing or if we simply desire more and more things to try and fill a void within us.

The late Wayne Dyer, in his book "Manifest your Destiny" says,

"The nature of gratitude helps us dispel the idea that we do not have enough and that we ourselves are not enough. When your heart is filled with gratitude it is grateful for everything and cannot focus on what is missing."

Wise words.

The more I develop my own grateful attitude each day the less I find I have to complain about!

Why practice gratitude?

Usui's precept asks us to live with appreciation. Why should we be grateful and appreciative? What difference can it make to our lives?

Research has shown that grateful people are actually happier in general than those who are ungrateful.

Think about it this way – if your house was burning down or if you only had moments to live – what would be important to you? Would it be the stuff you have accumulated?

I think not!

It is more likely to be the people in your life, your memories and your love that is important not the 52" flat screen on the wall or the shiny car in the driveway.

Developing an attitude of gratitude reminds us of what is important in life. It helps us to focus on the positives – on our blessings. It also helps us to turn negatives into positives.

For example – if you have had a rough day at work, at least you have a job to pay the bills and at least that day is over now and you are home safe and sound. Problems often help us grow as a person.

I read a lovely analogy of this on social media the other day. A man was sitting in his garden when he noticed a cocoon on one of the plants nearby.

As he watched he could see a tiny opening and from this opening a butterfly was struggling to emerge. He watched and waited patiently as the butterfly struggled and strained against the restrictive cocoon, trying to free itself.

After some time the butterfly stopped struggling and appeared to be beaten. The man was worried and thought he should help so he went inside and got a pair of scissors. He carefully snipped off part of the cocoon to allow the butterfly to emerge easily.

However he was shocked to see that the butterfly's body was very swollen and its wings were shrivelled and small. The butterfly emerged from the cocoon but was unable to fly – it spent the rest of its life crawling about.

In his kindness the man had prevented the full development of the creature. The point of the restrictive opening and struggle was to force liquid from the body of the butterfly into its wings thus enabling it to fly when it finally emerged.

And so it is for humans too – often our struggles are what makes us grow and we need them in order to learn and develop.

By developing an attitude of gratitude we can begin to see the bigger picture when struggles come our way and we can remain positive in the face of adversity.

Putting it into practice

So how do you actually begin to live with gratitude?

It is really quite easy – you begin by saying "Thank you". When someone does something for you, thank them. Why not thank the bus driver for driving you to your destination or thank the shop assistant for serving you?

When was the last time you sent a thank you card to someone?

Or the last time you rang or emailed someone to say thank you?

These days we have forgotten the joy of receiving a card in the post as everything is online – why not send a thank you card the next time someone gives you a gift or does something kind for you?

Have a morning and evening gratitude session. Each morning be thankful that you have woken up and that you have another day of life ahead of you – so many people don't! Be thankful for your body and the wonderful things it does for you to keep you alive.

In the evening, write down 5 things that you are grateful for that day. They don't have to be massive things – look at the simple things – thank you for the lady who held the door open for me in the shop, thank you for the sunshine today, thank you for the clean water I have from my tap, and so on.

I keep a gratitude journal and it really helps me when I find myself falling into a dark mood.

Each evening I write down 5 things from the day that I am thankful for – I try not to repeat myself each day so that by the end of the week and then the end of the month I have a lot to be thankful for. I read it back to myself every now and then and really count my blessings. Try it – it really works!

Why not try a simple exercise now – list your blessings.

How empty would your life be without your friends, family, home, everyday objects, etc.?

Take a moment to list all the things and people in your life that you are grateful for. Can you see how that helps to shift your focus from what you don't have to what you do have?

To develop an attitude of gratitude means to be willing to express appreciation to those you care about.

Say "I love you" more often. Thank them, give them gifts, and care for them.

Practice random acts of kindness. Do something for someone with no expectation of receiving anything in return. For example buy someone's coffee or pay it forward and leave money for the next person to come along. Hold a door open for someone or help an elderly person with their shopping or across the road.

When you notice that you are about to complain, stop yourself and pause. Most people are simply trying to do their best – look at the bigger picture before starting to complain.

Look at all the "things" you own – your home, your furniture, your gadgets, your food etc. All these things you owe to other people – those who built it or grew it, those who shipped it, those who distributed it and sold it.

Think about the food on your table – thank the earth for providing it, thank the farmer for tending the crops, thank the distributors for getting it out to the supermarkets, thank your boss for the job which allowed you to pay for the food, thank the person who manufactured your cooker so you could cook the food ... it's amazing when you start to think this way. It reminds us that we are all connected and that a little gratitude goes a really long way!

The next time you have to pay a bill, rather than grumbling about it, say thank you! You have the means to pay it and you are paying with a grateful heart for the service or utility you have received.

Give as generously as possible for the more generous of spirit you are the more you will find to be grateful for.

I hope that I have shown how developing an attitude of gratitude can benefit your life. When working with the Reiki principles it is so much more than simply meditating on them and chanting them morning and night. You actually have to live them and make them part of your everyday life – that is where the real magic and healing lies!

Chapter 15: Reiki For Stress Relief

Below are tips for reducing stress with Reiki:

1. Get situated

Turn your phone off and eliminate all other distractions. Sit upright in a position that is comfortable to you, or perhaps lie down if that is more suitable to you. If there is a time limit to how long you can practice, set an alarm clock ahead of time.

2. Get Centred

Place the hands over the eyes, and breathe in gently and let the air circulate to the abdomen. Take a deep breath in, hold it in for a couple moments, and then exhale. Repeat this several times. This exercise restores strained eyes and heals headaches. To help with an overactive or aroused mind, place the hands over the temples.

3. Releasing Tension

Move the hands to the rear part of the head or neck. This refreshes the brain and thereby releases a great deal of tension.

4. Focusing on the Neck

Moving the hands to the sides of the neck controls the thyroid, and also helps with communication.

5. Chest Area

Place the hands above the chest to aid in drainage of the lymph organs, and to help with purifying the body of toxins.

6. Heart Chakra

Placing the hands over the sternum bones helps in restoration of emotional health.

7. Navel

To centre yourself and balance out the entire Reiki process, finish with the hands just below the navel area.

8. Reintegrate

As your Reiki session comes to an end, slowly open the eyes. Soak it all in by staying quiet for a few moments, and remembering all you are thankful for in your life.

Extra Benefits

The medical industry discovers many new discoveries nearly every day. Some are promising, and some are found to be untrue later, and still others are far too costly for the average care-seeker to even consider. The discovery of Reiki by those looking for help is often a blessing, as it promises relief and help without much cost. Reiki is an ancient Asian art form, as stated before, but it is quickly gaining notoriety in much of the Western world, especially in younger generations. Even athletes are turning to Reiki to help with their injuries that naturally come with sports. The healing time has been generously cut down for many athletes who use the compounding power of Reiki along with standard rehabilitation methods.

Furthermore, breakthroughs are coming out regarding the use of Reiki in AIDS patients. AIDS has been the cause of a great amount of misery to many patients, but Reiki has been reported to bring positive energy into the patients' bodies, relieving some of their pain.

Since physically being with your patient is not always possible, distance healing is also becoming a popular form of Reiki. The relief is reported to be just as effective when patients encounter distance healing, and is more convenient for practitioners to be able to help clients all over the world.

Even pets are benefiting from the positive energy produced by Reiki. Veterinary costs are always going up, so this style is favoured because of its economic advantage, as well as being non-invasive and gentler for your beloved pet. Also, the calm movements do not stress the pet, as the uncomfortable positions that animal care professionals force the pet into, typically do.

Reiki provides leverage necessary for combating the underlying health problems that cause diseases. The underlying health condition is often a mental defect, and the transference of the positive energy into the mind often helps with any mental problem an individual has.

Reiki is recommended for pregnant ladies, as well. The complete experience of pregnancy is often more positive when Reiki is used. The positive energy around the pregnant mother ensures the health of the infant. Healthy and happy babies are a by-product of practicing Reiki while pregnant.

Many illnesses today need some type of invasive treatment. This further increases the anxiety in an individual who is diagnosed with a health condition. An introduction to any non-invasive technique can be quite comforting to the patient. This is undoubtedly part of the reason for Reiki's success.

Reiki touts many other benefits as well. Reiki has been known to increase blood simulation, which helps to stop bleeding in minor wounds. There have also been reports of purification of the arteries, liver, spleen, lungs and gall bladder. Nosebleeds, insomnia and depression have all also been cured with the help of Reiki. The recovery time after treatments is shortened. Best of all, there is no pain caused by Reiki, contrary to the treatments done by the modern medical industry, which are typically painful or at least have undesirable side effects in some way. In fact, it is so comfortable that some people even report dozing off during a Reiki session.

Without trying Reiki, one will never know the recovery that may have been possible or how much easier rehabilitation could have been. Regular practice of Reiki is recommended to increase the mental state, and hence, the positivity of your outlook of life. The more positive you look at your daily situations, the happier you will be in life.

Getting the Most out of Reiki

Practice Any Time

You can practice Reiki on yourself at any time of day. Many people like to start their day with Reiki, which prepares them for their whole day. Others prefer ending their days with Reiki, which helps with relaxation and unwinding so they get a good night's sleep. A complete hour of Reiki healing is ideal, but if this is not possible, a simple 15 to 20 minutes also serves a useful purpose and can benefit you daily.

Practice on a Regular Basis

Gaining the skills it takes to master Reiki takes much time and many attempts on your part. Commitment of time and perseverance with practicing the skills are imperative when trying to master this art form. In today's fast paced environment, it is often a challenge in itself to be able to delay gratification and take the time it takes to learn new skills. It is to be expected that Reiki take several months or even up to a year of practice before results can be seen.

The negative side effects that come with medical conditions are usually just deemed as necessary evils. These side effects often increase the stress that the patient originally had about the medical condition, which can escalate recovery time significantly. Reiki can help patients with the side effects of their treatments, thereby increasing recovery rate, decreasing needed medications, and reducing tension in the patient's life in general.

It is worth noting that an open and positive outlook about Reiki can greatly enhance your results with it. The recipient's willingness to explore Reiki and positive mentality is essential to the success of Reiki.

Flow of Energy

To understand the flow of energy, it is helpful to imagine the energy as a tangible object. For instance, envision that the energy is a golden flowing object, and that it is streaming into the body from the hands, circulating the wounded body part, and nourishing each cell, tissue and organ that needs and craves it. Let your hands rest at the wounded area for as long as it is comfortable. You may notice the body part receiving the energy begin to get warmer and warmer.

Commitment to the Reiki Process

Staying committed to Reiki, helps the body rid itself of pollutants, and maintains the positive effects it brings to the emotions, mind and entire body. Staying committed to a weekly ritual will help you realise the potential of Reiki.

Other Tips

Getting the most out of Reiki takes preparation and alteration of lifestyles. The first suggestion is to consume a vegetarian diet, and to stop consuming alcohol, drugs and any toxins such as those from pesticide residue. Sweets and cigarettes are also not conducive to achieving all the effects Reiki can offer. These ingredients work against Reiki, as Reiki's ultimate goal is purity, and these substances throw the system off balance, making the smooth flow of Reiki difficult or even impossible. If these materials cannot be completely eliminated from your life, try to remove them for at least a few days before your Reiki session.

A calm lifestyle can also help enhance your Reiki results. This is hard in current times, with the media constantly reporting negative stories, increasing stress levels and even blood pressure. Also, jobs and extra-curricular activities keep the majority of people extremely busy. However, if possible, cutting out detrimental TV programmes, movies, video games and violent music will contribute to the gaining of purity in life that Reiki helps to maintain.

Some highly devoted Reiki followers even go so far as to cut off contact with people who they feel have negative energy. They feel this negative energy can affect their own lives, and do not want to be connected to such undesirable forces.

This guide should enlighten you about the practice of Reiki. Many have found it helpful, and hopefully it can bring some peace into your life. Good luck with your quest to find your own brand of Reiki!

Chapter 16: A Simple Meditation.

Much has been written about meditation and many strange ideas exist. This is a simple meditation that is easy to lean and to practice. It has helped me and I feel can benefit most of us. In the hustle and bustle of modern life it is increasingly difficult to find peace and quiet. Our minds are constantly on the go. Even when we are supposedly relaxing it is all too easy to be involved in tomorrow's work or analysing what has happened earlier.

It is important therefore to give ourselves a real break to allow our minds to "take a deep breath and relax". In this way we can see things clearly and not in the reflection of our hectic lives.

Try and give yourself ten to fifteen minutes in the morning and evening to practice this meditation.

I also like to use it to prepare myself before I treat patients. It makes for a calm and restful treatment and allows me easier access to my intuition.

Gassho Meditation.

Gassho is the Japanese word for "two hands

 (are) coming together".

Sit in what ever position you feel comfortable, either on the floor cross legged or in a chair, but try and keep the spine straight. (There is nothing wrong with lying down or leaning against something the only trouble is that it is very easy to doze off).

Take a few deep breaths to relax yourself and close your eyes. Take a couple more deep breaths just to settle things down a bit. Now bring your hands together in a praying position in front of you heart.

Bring your attention to the point where the middle fingers of both hands touch and focus it there. The idea is to concentrate all your attention solely on the touching of these two fingers and to allow all other thoughts to cease to exist. This is jolly near impossible and almost immediately your mind will bounce off on some thought or other. Gently observe the thought; let it go and return to focusing on your two fingers. Each time your mind wanders treat it in the same way, neither judging nor criticising your success or lack of it. The point of this meditation is the doing not an end result.

Chapter 17: More Advantages Of Reiki

Synopsis

Reiki is an ancient form of harnessing positive energy from one source and transferring it on to another, for healing purposes.

Practicing reiki brings many advantages into an individual's life. The more popularly and common benefits from practicing reiki are; relief from mental and physical stress, relaxation, comfort in body and mind and surroundings and peace, to name a few.

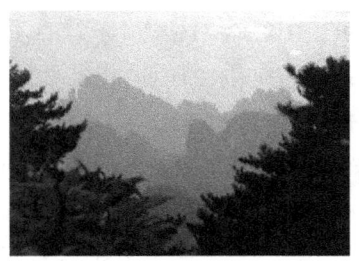

A Few More Advantages

There are also other little known advantages to practicing reiki, though none any less beneficial. Some reiki practitioners practice this art form to induce spiritual clarity. In offering the relief needed during emotional distress and sorrow, reiki helps one be more connected to the center of one's spirituality, thus preventing the state of mind and body to feel totally drained.

Reiki also works to relief pain while improving the general blood circulation throughout the body. In doing so, reiki can also contribute to hastening the stoppage of small bleeding wounds. Some reiki practitioners also attest to the benefits of the cleansing element reiki can effect in the liver, arteries, spleen, gall bladder, and lungs. There are many other illnesses or ailment the reiki has been found to play a positive role when introduced as a complimenting therapy to ongoing medical procedures or medications. Some of these medical conditions have to be endured with considerable pain before reiki was introduced, to bring the much needed relief, at least from the pain enduring angle.

Some medical conditions are generally linked to some kind of imbalance and reiki has also made positive in road in the area. Medical conditions such as chronic and acute nose bleeds, chronic insomnia, depression, menopause to name a few are where reiki has been a positive benefit. Reiki has also been known to be used to speed up the recovery process after surgery. The positive energy transference helps to bring about a positive and quick recovery, without the use of further adding on any medications.

Chapter 18: Energeticbodies

THE AURA—THE SUBTLE BODY

Quantum physics describes the universe as energy, with energy and matter interchangeable. Psychology, Eastern therapy, and complementary medicine all have terms for life as energy. The aura can be viewed as an energy field surrounding the body, interacting through spiritual and psychological levels via structures called chakras. In other words, the aura is an energy field that surrounds the physical body, discernible to those of psychical sight.

Attunements strengthen the aura throughout one's life from 6-11 feet.

The seven main chakras have their origin in the physical body but they also exist in all the layers of the aura. The speed and vibration level of the energy is increased with each level. Human consciousness is imprinted into the seven layers that constitute the aura.

How Reiki Affects The Aura

Before a Reiki attunement a person's aura may only extend a few inches to a foot outside the person's body. Attunements strengthen the aura throughout one's life from 6-11 feet. Also, one's inner strength and intuition act as a guide to facilitate change and increase optimum health. Through the strengthening of the aura, many aspects of your life improve.

During a Reiki treatment, the organs and energy flow within the body affected, as well as various bodies of the aura. When using distance healing or the mental/emotional symbol, the aura seems to be more affected than the actual organs in the body.

The Different Layers/Bodies In The Aura

The Physical body is the most tangible manifestation of our consciousness. Its function is to be here and now. We act consciously: being present when walking, enjoying our food when eating, etc.
The Etheric body is a 3 inch thin invisible layer around the physical body. This is where the energy is reflected when it flows through meridians and chakras. This acts as a template for the physical body and appears as an energy matrix. Chinese medicine describes this as meridians that transmit Chi (Ki) through the body. It is in this body that we feel the sensations of physical pleasure or pain.

Many of our dreams can be found in the etheric body. Mantras, symbols and essences can affect this part of the aura. It is connected to the root chakra.

The Emotional body is the third body. It is egg-shaped and contains the physical and etheric bodies. This body reflects our feelings and emotions, such as happiness, hope, love, anger, sorrow and hate. It is also connected to our past, which can cause problems. The body is cocooned by desires from the past, which sometimes cause tension. It is important to learn how to handle different emotions throughout the day; the risk is they become suppressed and stored in the emotional body and later cause blockages and disturbances, leading to medical problems. It is connected to the navel chakra.

The Mental body teaches us self-knowledge. It reflects the conscious mind, logic, intellect and active thinking.

We shape our reality with our minds. It is the builder. It reflects our ability wherein which we develop our learning and personality. Mental health or mental illness is reflected in this body. It is connected to the solar plexus chakra.

The Astral body is the bridge between the physical world and the spiritual realm. It represents unconditional love and a connection to the heart chakra.

The Etheric Template body (Divine Will) can be identified with memory and our thought processes. It also stores the present and all possible future probabilities. It is connected to the throat chakra.

The Celestial body mirrors the subconscious mind that is a part of the inactive part of our brain. By listening to your subconscious, your intuition, your journey through life is more simple and rewarding. Expressed within this body is unconditional love, a universal love for all life. It is connected to the third-eye point/chakra.

The Causal body (Ketheric Template) is the last body. The energies in this body spin at a very high frequency. This is where the soul communicates with the conscious mind via the subconscious mind in the mental body. The initial creative impulse begins here. It goes beyond linear knowing into an integrated knowing. It is connected to the crown chakra.

Reiki increases your energy, rather than depleting you when giving treatments.

Treatments

HANDS TRANSMITTING ENERGY

Palms: Healing Vessels

Your palms are vessels giving forth the Reiki energy. The selftreatments nourish and sensitize you to feeling the subtle differences of energy flow that emanate through your hands. Remember, Reiki is derived from an infinite source. Therefore, it increases your energy level, rather than depleting you when you give treatments. You are now becoming a purer Reiki conduit. You will need self-compassion for proper rest and to treat yourself regularly. This does require a relaxed yet disciplined approach to honor different body parts/chakras with 1-5 minute dosages of hands-on self treatments.

Once past your 21-day cleansing period, a weekly full body treatment will surpass any spa treatment. I refer to this as my Soul Spa Treatment (This option is offered to clients seeking deeper rejuvenation. It puts one into a very blissful state where you are communing with the Divine.) Just imagine! You have said yes to receiving through your own self treatments. You create an instant connection with Source energy. It responds through your healing vessels—the hands which extend from the heart and Divine love.

No Flow?

You may question if there is "enough" coming through your hands or if the sensations in your palms are weak, not warm enough or cold. The more you use Reiki, the more you recognize various sensations in your hands, heart and third-eye point. Simply by placing your hands on a person is the signal for switching the energy on regardless of your conscious awareness.

Experiencing the flow of energy is individual. Self-healing treatments assist in aligning yourself with the energy. Taking this meditative time familiarizes you with how the energy flows

You have received the attunements to access a limitless and abundant life force. The Creator dwells within this; it IS the energy working through you.

through you. (This is what the 4th precept emphasizes: **"Today, I do my work honestly."** It underlies a daily spiritual and meditation practice for contemplation and awareness of Reiki).

When treating others, ask for their feedback to build your confidence. Sometimes, you may overanalyze and become anxious that something is **wrong** with you. Honor the adjustment period to recognize energy sensations.

Patience and compassion apply to accessing Reiki. Trust that the energy is flowing appropriately to the situation, physical body part, or particular emotion, etc. You have received the attunements to access a limitless and abundant life force. The Creator dwells within this; it **is** the energy working **through** you.

REIKI ON THE GO

Already knowing the proper sequence from self-practice, you can also send Reiki to any aspects of your life that require change or clarity. Envision the first Reiki symbol, Cho Ku Rei, you have been introduced to. See it penetrating that person's aura, situation or circumstance you are dealing with. Again, your intention is a strong and powerful tool.

You can also tune into Reiki while doing chores, studying, sitting in car traffic or on public transportation, waiting your turn in line. In bureaucratic dealings in court or DMV, I have sent Reiki to the four corners of the room, to the highest good of the situation, and directly to the person dealing with me—aiming it at their heart from my heart center. I bless my mail before opening or play with Reiki by holding the envelopes between my palms and during phone calls with customer service. Even in meetings, if I am called to calm anyone—I send Reiki to them. When my solar plexus or any chakra needs energizing, I discreetly rest my palms there and secretly bliss out! Wherever you go, Reiki is with you!

Self-Treatment

HEAL YOURSELF, HEAL THE WORLD

Reiki is a system comprised of specific elements that essentially raises YOUR life force energy. Dr. Usui began his teachings as a spiritual practice for himself. He realized the ultimate healing tool is self-practice—a dedication to heal the Self. Only then were these techniques passed on to others.

This is an example of beginning the healing journey with and within ourselves. We make ourselves "healthy, happy and (w)holly" by venturing within. We become the change that we want to see in the world. This affects everyone and everything around us.

To be effective healers, we need to heal ourselves.

Self-practice is the essence of Reiki.

To be effective healers, we need to heal ourselves. It is essential It is essential day cleansing period, extending up to 30 days.

This helps you to adjust to the new energy you have accepted and assists you in becoming a clearer Reiki channel. The peace which moves through you is truly magnificent. (Based on my personal experiences, I easily "bliss out" into a holistic paradise and need a timer to pull me back to earth where time does not stand still!)

It is this state of tranquility that carries over into your day so you are able to recognize negative thoughts and habits. This allows you to change your belief patterns—those mental emotional grooves created long ago which get deeper each time your "monkey mind" revisits them. I assure you, regular selftreatments act as an overall preventative "dis-ease" measure. Since that brings a sense of well-being, it reduces stress and has a positive, calming effect on all aspects of your life—including those cute monkeys that thrive to wreak havoc in your mind. (Remember to affirm **The Five Precepts!**)

Feed yourself love and re-gain control of your life—a life that is worthy to be fully lived in joy. You will even move into more non-reactive states of being and be less likely to react

It is this state of tranquility that carries over into your day so you are able to recognize negative thoughts and habits. As the energy stimulates the cells and molecules, your body adjusts and relaxes into its natural original state of harmonious balance.

negatively to difficult situations. Therefore, self-practice is the essence of the Reiki teachings.

As you relax, ALLOW yourself to be receptive and **divinely irresistible** to Reiki, it gradually leads you toward your heart's center—the center of all things, and **honu**

no reiko, the spiritual light within. It is a path to personal and spiritual growth where you deepen the connection to **dwelling in possibility**—dwelling in Divine Love.

CREATE A SACRED SPACE

Create a comfortable, relaxing environment in a room where you enjoy the energy. Ideally, create an altar with a few favorite spiritual items. This will set and keep a higher vibrational tone for you. Allow for uninterrupted time—early morning or evening, preferably the same time every day. The selftreatments may be very relaxing for you or energizing. Take this into account when choosing your time preference.

Dwell in possibility.
 Dwell in Divine love!

Turn your phones off. Tell others to leave you alone without distractions. Keep a blanket nearby as your body temperature may drop. Relaxing meditative music, a pillow, clock or cell phone alarm that rings every two-five minutes are all useful (to signal switching to the next body position). Remember, it is easy to lose track of time and fall into a semi-conscious sleep (a signal that a specific area is depleted and drawing a bigger dose of energy).

As the energy stimulates the cells and molecules, your body adjusts and relaxes into its natural original state of harmonious balance. For this reason, many people avoid treatments lying down. Find your personal preference by practicing various methods. Ultimately, the alarm signals the end and you slowly re-enter the world revitalized.

BEGIN WITH AN INTENTION

To make the most of your self-treatment, it is beneficial to set a positive intent for each personal session. This is your sacred moment. Make the most of it by honing in on grander, healthier visions. Your general intention/Reiki prayer can be

"Thank you Reiki for gracefully working in and through me. May this treatment benefit

me and may I be a conduit of service." **stated simply,** "Thank you Reiki for gracefully working in and through me. May this treatment benefit me. May I be a conduit of service."

You can be specific if that is more comforting. It is what you are being guided to say and experience in that moment. However you word it, by releasing the intent for the highest good of all concerned, you are detaching from the outcome, you trust that the Reiki intelligence has your best intentions in the heart of the Universe.

After 21 days of consistently practicing self-treatments, you will have grown accustomed to the proper sequence of hand positions, the various sensations that emanate from your palms, and how it is felt within your body.

From this time forward, you will be more adept at recognizing areas of your body that are calling out for a deeper healing. You can now direct and focus your hands on the area in need, bypassing the learned sequence. However, it is beneficial to keep up with full body treatments. This is a great way to remain tuned up and plugged into higher states of awareness. You will notice a difference if you stop the self-treatments for a few days and then begin again. I warmly and emphatically urge you to set aside self-healing time. This will become an enjoyable established blissful routine!

REVEALING FOR HEALING

The intention you set can lead you into a conversation with that particular body part, organ or emotion. As Reiki begins to move within you, a deep sense of peace is attained. You relax into the energy and give up any resistance to messages from your inner being and whatever is calling out to be loved. You connect on a sublime Divine level to this particular area that is revealing to you an imbalance: **a shortage of love**.

Healing is a letting go of fear. It is surrendering those fears to a Higher Power. Acknowledgment of that Divine Higher Presence is accepting love (which annihilates fear—zaps it on the spot!) and creates **"peace that passeth all understanding."** Ultimate optimum health stems from that serene, tranquil state.

As Reiki begins to move within you, a deep sense of peace is attained. Ultimate optimum health stems from that serene, tranquil state. Spend approximately 3-5 minutes on each position, unless you feel a pull of energy or extra tingling in your palms

Yes, each miniscule part of you has a voice that awaits to reveal itself to you. When you are not loving those disconnected parts and your Self due to harboring doubts, fears and negativities, you constrict the flow of loving kindness, compassion and abundance into your life.

THE ACTUAL TREATMENT

When giving yourself a Reiki treatment, consider using comfortable pillows to position under your arms or back.

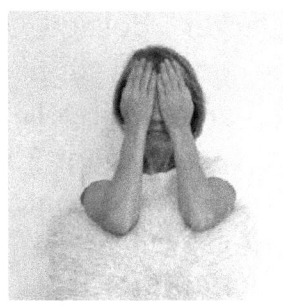

Keep contact with your body while changing hand positions since the energy becomes restricted if the deep relaxation is interrupted. Lying down or sitting in a chair allows you to reach all the positions. Many of the self-treatment positions shown below are sitting. This seems to be most comfortable for those that need a quick pick-me-up during the day or to fall asleep. You can vary your treatments sitting or lying down to alter your experiences.

Spend approximately 2-5 minutes on each position, unless you feel there is a pull of energy or extra tingling in your palms. This is a signal that this area is more depleted, requiring a larger dosage of energy. Remain in the position until the hands stop buzzing or intuitively you feel complete. Mrs. Takata spent 30 minutes in one hand position if that area was suffering. In your state of tranquility, you will be receptive to wisdom from your Higher Self. You will know when to move onto the next position.

Mrs. Takata spent 30 minutes on troubled areas.

Generally, your fingers and thumbs are held together. This allows for a freer flow of energy. David Vennells in his book, **Beginner's Guide to Reiki**, explains that the second (index finger) and longest finger (the middle Saturn finger) stimulate the palm chakras. He suggests massaging the palms in a circular motion. You can also draw a counterclockwise spiral in the air above them or right onto each palm with the index and middle fingers. A movement of energy may be felt within the palm. Reiki attunements sensitize your palms due to the increase of life force energy it has created within you.

The index and middle fingers stimulate the palm chakras.

After your 21-day cleansing period when you have befriended the energy, felt the effects and become more adept, you can add additional stimuli with crystals and/or aromatherapy to enhance your relaxation and wellness.

Your in-between treatments can be 20 minutes total. When you need to conserve time, choose three positions you are most drawn to and stay with each for five minutes.

Chapter 19: Attunement - All Degrees

These are the attunements that have been handed down and should never be altered. Add to them but **"always in addition too, never instead of."**

Method

1) Have the recipient(s) sit in a chair with their feet uncrossed and planted on the floor with their hands together in front of them.

2) Stand in front of and facing the person(s) with your hands together, and say to them "When you feel my hands on your head, assume the prayer position", and show them the prayer position with your hands.

 (Say this only once, whether you are attuning one or more people.)

3) Ask (all of) the recipient(s) to close their eyes.

4) Stand in front of the (first) recipient.

5) Walk **counter-clockwise** around the first person and stand behind them.

6) Stand briefly behind with your hands together while you connect to the Earth and silently ask for help and support from the Circle of Reiki Masters.

7) Contract your Hui Yin by clenching you buttocks and place the tip of your tongue on the roof of your mouth (see First Degree book – Steppe 1). This allows a flow around the spine and brain energy paths.

8) Gently place both your hands on the top of the recipient's head for a count of nine heartbeats. Tune into the recipient's soul. Allow yourself to come into deep relation in your heart.

9) Remove both of your hands. You may want to place your non-dominant hand on your solar plexus or hara. This is for your protection or comfort.

10) Using your dominant hand, draw the **Dai Koo Myo** symbol horizontally over the person's head **once, twice or thrice** with the palm of your hand whilst silently saying the symbol name to yourself **three** times and visualising the symbol in violet.

11) Follow the same process as step 10 with **Choku Rei**.

12) Gently place your dominant hand on the recipient's head and visualise the **Hon Sha Ze Sho Nen** in violet - you may draw it instead if you wish - while repeating the symbol name to yourself **three** times.

13) Visualise - or draw - the **Sei He Ki** in violet while saying the symbol name to yourself **three** times.

14) Remove your hand from the recipient's head and walk counter-clockwise to the front of the chair so you are facing the recipient. The recipient's hands should be in the prayer position. If not, gently reposition them.

15) Take the recipient's hands with your non-dominant hand (from the front or the back), position them in front of their heart and touch their fingertips with the fingertips of your dominant hand.

16) Continue to hold the recipient's hands during steps 17 to 28 with your non-dominant hand.

17) With your dominant hand, draw the **Dai Koo Myo once, twice** or **thrice** horizontally over the recipient's fingertips, while visualising it in violet and saying the symbol name to yourself **three** times.

18) Follow the same process in step 17 for steps 18-20 with the different symbols. **Choku Rei**.

19) Hon Sha Ze Sho Nen.

20) Sei He Kei.

21) Visualise the **Dai Koo Myo** very clearly in violet, say the name silently to yourself and blow it into the recipient's fingertips.

22) Position the recipient's hands up so their fingertips are about one inch above their third eye (Sixth Chakra).

23) With your dominant hand, draw the **Dai Koo Myo once, twice** or **thrice** horizontally over the recipient's fingertips, while visualising it in violet and saying the symbol name to yourself **three** times.

24) Follow the same process in step 23 for steps 24-26 with the different symbols. **Choku Rei**.

25) Hon Sha Ze Sho Nen.

26) Sei He Kei.

27) Visualise the **Dai Koo Myo** very clearly in violet, say the name silently to yourself, and blow out across their fingertips, upward through the point on the forehead opposite their fingertips and toward their crown chakra.

28) Separate the recipient's hands and move them towards their lap. As you do so, press your thumbs into their palms to begin activation of their hand chakras. Position their hands with their palms facing up.

29) Release the recipient's hands.

30) Hold the recipient's right hand, palm up, with your non-dominant hand. Draw

the **Choku Rei** with your dominant palm over their palm and slap it into their hand. Release their right hand.

31) Repeat step 30 for the recipient's left hand.

32) Bring their hands together in a prayer position, move them up so the base of their thumbs touches their third eye, visualise the **Dai Koo Myo** clearly in your third eye in violet, say the name silently to yourself and blow it across their fingertips and across their crown, front to back.

33) Lower the recipient's hands to the front of their heart in a prayer position. Remove your hands and touch them to the ground in front of the recipient. Give an appropriate silent prayer or blessing.

34) Step back from the recipient. Silently bow.

35) If you are attuning more than one person, stand in front of the next person and start their attunement. When you have completed the last attunement, give a blessing to the whole group and gently let them know that their attunements are complete.

36) Handing them a Reikied glass of water is very grounding and pleasant.

37) Respect the need for some to remain silent whilst others may need to talk.

A reminder: If You Make a Mistake During an Attunement...

If, for instance, you do not draw a symbol correctly, stop drawing the symbol, pump your Hui Yin **three** times, and redraw the symbol from the beginning. You do not need to start the entire sequence of symbols over, only the one you were drawing when the error occurred. As you re-draw the symbol, remember to say the name silently **three** times.

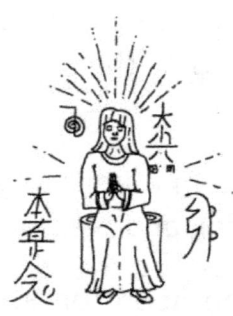

Generating and Administering Classes

Working with other teachers is a positive way to start giving Reiki attunements

Brain storming ideas and generating new growth keeps the teaching fresh and alive. Work at your own pace with an open and loving heart so miracles will surely follow.

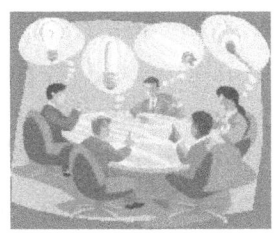

A good friend said:

"Time tables and written speeches/sermons are like lifeboats, to be launched in times of emergencies".

Get to know your routine well enough so you use it as a check list if needed. However, we are enclosing the teaching plans that have been tried and tested by many as a basis for your own creativity.

It is said a good teacher is one that is prepared enough so it **seems** everything is spontaneous. In some case the attunements **will** become totally spontaneous so do get familiar enough with them to do them when required unexpectedly. Above all remember Reiki attunements, as Reiki healing, comes **through** you not **from** you. If you drift off to another plane it will still happen anyway.

Tell the participants

What you are going to do

Do it

Tell them what you have done

The places used and the number of participants can be as varied as the numbers interested in healing generally. Do be flexible and allow the Higher Intelligence to lead you through if you begin to doubt. In the wider scheme of things remember all is perfect, whole and complete **just as it is now**.

Teacher's plans, posters, application forms, confirmation of classes etc. are available but we encourage you to be creative and develop your own literature as you develop other skills.

Now you have accepted the gift of Reiki attuning

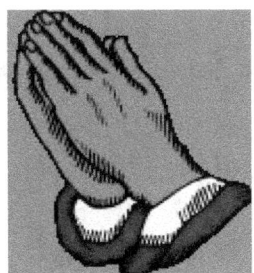

Guidelines for your Integration Period

o   Meditate each day for at least 15 minutes with no energy work and no agenda.

o   Treat yourself daily with Reiki as you prepare for sleep, upon waking and other times during the day.

o Treat someone with Reiki at a distance each day.

o Do Reiki attunements each day on a partner, stuffed animal, or imaginary friend.

o Keep a daily journal of written and / or drawn expressions of your feelings about Reiki, your progress with attunements, feelings of readiness to teach and anything else that comes up in your personal process that relates to receiving the Initiation.

Write to your attuner in 21 days summarising the journal and addressing the following questions and sharing anything you would like to with them

1) What does it mean to you to be a teacher of Reiki?

2) How has your life changed since you made the decision to take on this next

step in your development as a Healer and Teacher?

3) What is your experience of the energy? Is it different than before trying Attunements?

4) How do you see yourself using Reiki in your life's mission?

5) What is your greatest dream of enlightened service?

Keep closely in touch with others in the Reiki family.

We all need each other's support in these changing times. There may be times of difficulty, frustration and problems ahead. With love and understanding, we will grow stronger together. A healer in every home? Of course!!!

Often just *being* instead of *doing* is most effective with any healing and Reiki in particular. Have fun and enjoy your attunements.

Wishing you love, blessings and warm hands always.

Chapter 20: Meditation

In this chapter, there are some meditations that you can try. There are lots of different types of meditation. Some schools of Reiki encourage meditation to help with your personal growth, wellbeing and spirituality. It can also help you develop your skills as a Reiki practitioner. Here are some other benefits of meditating: -

BENEFITS OF MEDITATION

-Helps with energy levels.

-Helps you to see things with clarity, from an objective point of view.

-Helps you cope and deal with situations.

-Helps you cope and deal with negative or strong emotions.

-Encourages relaxation, both in the short term and long term.

-Develops tolerance and patience.

-Encourages you to live in the moment, rather than in the past (depression) or the future (anxiety).

-Can help with anxiety, addiction, and other mental health problems (but also seek professional advice and support).

-Can help with pain and health problems.

-Can help you to solve problems.

-Ability to look at, discover and potentially change your thought patterns.

-Boosts the immune system.

-Aids creativity.

-Helps with self-confidence and self-esteem.

-Can cure headaches and migraines.

-Can help with sleep problems.

-It is said to help improve sense of humour!

-It can be used as a spiritual practice and spiritual growth, or just simply for health reasons.

-And many more...!

MEDITATION TIPS

- Find a meditation that works best for you. There are plenty of meditation classes available. There are lots of other meditations available that I haven't included.

- Similar to Reiki, meditation can be spiritual or non-spiritual (just simply for health and relaxation reasons).

- Meditation is a way of quieting/relaxing the mind (NOT emptying it). We do this by focusing our attention on one single object, chant/words or sensation. You can also do walking meditations, chi kung, tai chi or yoga.

- Your attention will probably drift and become wrapped up in your thoughts or other distractions. When this happens, acknowledge it and simply bring your focus back to your meditation (without policing it or being hard on yourself).

-Make sure your meditation is not too loose or too rigid (both body and mind are comfortable and relaxed, but the meditation still remains focused and alert, i.e. without falling asleep).

-It's just a matter of regular practice (maybe even the same time each day).

-Enjoy the process, don't worry about the end result or police it (this is good, this is bad, I'm rubbish, I'll never do this!).

Here are just some meditations for you to try out.

DIAPHRAGM BREATHING

If you look at how babies breathe, you will see they actually breathe from their belly – their stomach goes up and down. As we grow older, we develop bad habits and start to breath from our chest. Short chest breathing is associated with all sorts of problems, including panic attacks, anxiety, breathing problems, aggravating asthma, and so on.

It is still healthy to do chest breathing (in a relaxed, healthy way) but we also need to do diaphragm breathing as it encourages the body to relax – it is linked to the parasympathetic nervous system.

-*Chest breathing* – encourages the sympathetic nervous system, which is the active part of our nervous system and provides air and oxygen to vital organs.

-*Diaphragm breathing* – encourages the parasympathetic nervous system, which helps us to relax and slow down.

-*Other types of breathing* – there are other breathing techniques in yoga.

Gently breathe in through your nose, but try and fill your stomach with air (the lower part of your rib cage). This is the bottom of your lungs and your diaphragm, which is a muscle.

Hold the breath in for as long as you can.

Gently breathe out.

Repeat as many times as you can.

It is important not to over breathe – it has to be a gentle natural process. It may be hard at first because we're not used to doing it – for that reason practice for short periods throughout the day e.g. during the adverts when a television program is on, or when you're waiting at red traffic lights for 1 minute.

Conclusion

In reality, nature is composed of simple elements. The apparent complexity of the universe is defined by the infinite interactions between these simple elements. Our attitude should imitate nature and seek simplicity. You will not get better results by complicating your techniques. Especially Reiki, which arises from nature itself, is an example of simplicity. When a person comes to you, offer him what you have. If that is not what he needs, it will be of no use to decorate or disguise it. In that case, the best thing you can do to do for that person is to allow him to continue the search for what he needs, without stopping him. The desire to improve is good, as it leads us to work and change for it. The need to offer better techniques led me to study acupuncture, which was one of the best things that happened to me. The problem can arise when we do not understand reality, and we pretend that we can get what we want without looking for it.

The desire to be recognized can lead us to want to be more than we are and to want to heal. Wanting to be recognized is part of our human nature. If you review the theory of the Chakras, in the bioenergetic manual, you will see that it is part of the third Chakra, Manipura. Being recognized as one of the forces that push us to find a place in society so that we are useful to those around us. The problem comes if this desire increases until we separate our mind from reality. So, instead of working on reality, on our attitudes, knowledge, and skills, in order to reach that goal (to be useful to others = to be recognized) we lose our way. When this happens we lose sight of the place where we are, and we pretend to be recognized before having found our place in society, something that goes against nature.

Our fears are the result of the desire to heal and the illusion of having in us the ability to do so. If we understand that the healing process does not depend on us, what reason is there to fear failure? If we limit ourselves to doing what we know how to do and we do it in the best possible way, there is no possible mistake. These fears are the result of the desire to be more than one is, to pretend to offer more than what we have. We only have to be afraid of if we appear what we are not and hide our reality from others, offering what we do not have. If we accept our limitations and show our resources and knowledge to others in an open way, as they are, it is not possible to live in fear.

Fear of reproaches is the result of the desire to be recognized, of the dependence on the judgments of others. It may be difficult to accept, but we will always be subject to the trials and reproaches of others, because "it never appeals to everyone's taste". Despite doing your job flawlessly, you will stumble upon people who will feel disappointed because they have not found in you what they hoped to find, or who will feel hurt because through you they have seen that part of themselves that they wish they had not seen.

Have you shown yourself as you are? Have you put all the cards on the table? In that case, you don't have to worry that someone has been disappointed. It was not you who let her down. Have you been kind and understanding? Have you always guided your conduct for righteousness and love for the person in front of you? Do not worry about your pain. It is the pain produced by the vision of reality that makes us wake up from the dream that separates us from the world. It has not been you who have hurt that person; she hurt herself by lying and falsifying her own reality.

The desires are born from a part of us that reminds us that we have not arrived at the place that corresponds to us and pushes us to walk to reach our place in this world. Fears are born of pretending to be better than what we are, of not understanding that in order to reach our goal we need to travel the path. It is necessary to walk but not forgetting where we are at each moment. If I fix my sight only at the end of the road, my consciousness and my intention will remain on the goal, but my steps will be insecure and I will constantly stumble. If I let the stumbling blocks and stones divert my attention, I will forget which path and where on the road I am.

We must keep an eye out to see where we are, and take care of the stumbling blocks we find along the way.

www.ingramcontent.com/pod-product-compliance
Lightning Source LLC
Chambersburg PA
CBHW052204090526
44583CB00015BA/1412

Justin Isis's previous works include "I Wonder What Human Flesh Tastes Like" (Chômu Press, 2011), "Welcome to the Arms Race" (Chômu Press, 2015), "Pleasant Tales II" (Snuggly Books, 2018) and the poetry collection "Divorce Procedures for the Hairdressers of a Metallic and Inconstant Goddess" (Snuggly Books, 2016). He also edited Chômu's "Dadaoism" anthology (2012), "Marked to Die: A Tribute to Mark Samuels" (Snuggly Books, 2016) and "Drowning in Beauty: The Neo-Decadent Anthology" (Snuggly Books, 2018). He currently lives in Tokyo.

JUSTIN ISIS

Instagrimoire//Fax Screen Sect: The Cancellation of Graham Greene, Volume 1: Tales from Orthographic Oceans, or: A Room with a View (Self-Portrait in a Concave Mirror with Interior Landscape & Key to the Scriptures)

THIS IS A SNUGGLY BOOK

Copyright © 2022 by Justin Isis.
All rights reserved.

ISBN: 978-1-64525-102-6

TABLE OF CONTENTS

PLATFORMAILURE / 9

THE TITANIC ANNOYANCE / 11

AGAINST VALENTINUS / 13

THE GHOST OF HANA KIMURA / 15

JASON, KING OF THE VAMPIRES / 20

THE TYRANNOSAUR OF TRADITION / 21

YOUR OTHER BODY / 24

THE GENERATIONS OF GRAHAM GREENE / 27

THE ACCREDITED GRAVE / 29

FACELESS RECOGNITION / 31

CAPITALIST CATECHISM / 33

SHIBUYA VS AKIHABARA / 34

POSTSCRIPT TO BRAUTIGAN / 36

ONLY TENTATIVELY DID I CANCEL GRAHAM GREENE / 38

DISQUALIFIED FROM BEING DISQUALIFIED FROM
    BEING HUMAN / 42

Instagrimoire//Fax Screen Sect: The Cancellation of Graham Greene, Volume 1: Tales from Orthographic Oceans, or: A Room with a View (Self-Portrait in a Concave Mirror with Interior Landscape & Key to the Scriptures)

PLATFORMAILURE

Unfollow yourself
like a shadow
slipping past perspective
in a de Chirico.

Ignore the influence
of pastel travel snaps
and all filtered lunches
of professional party guests:
fail to follow, friend or request.

Fail more
and even worse, for wear:
don't fail better
at the prospect of a purse
or any in-app purchase.

Escape before
some ivory-mouthed Rebecca
microdoses validation

in the corner of your attention
while tiny ugly dogs duplicate
beyond tolerance.

Wait for less marketable
emotions to arrive like cats
or other alienated majesties immodestly
falling to Earth and flashing
satanic smiles
of protracted languor
present in no
instant grammar.

THE TITANIC ANNOYANCE

Released from the rock
Prometheus found fire
was not enough for the freeloaders
and cargo cult kids demanding swag—
Strong AI and Frankenstein
eternal life and a leash for time
all loves requited and even
the real goods:
square triangles
a jailbroke genie
and the thing analogous to irony
with which the gods keep busy
through idle eternity.

And in return?
Poems and portraits
statues and sacrifices
keys to kingdoms
not worth the loss
of a liver.

In truth he'd never guessed the cost
of what had only been leftover fire
found in the couch
and scattered about in boredom—
"A bit like feeding the birds," he'd said.
"You like feeding birds?" They'd said.

Now the pilgrims
are clambering up his couch
and in his ire
he's sometimes thought
to gift them that perfect clock
counting down to the final human breath.
That, perhaps, would burn better than fire.
But why risk a return to the rock?

AGAINST VALENTINUS

Are these carceral embodiments,
matrices of phantom atoms
plotted by hidden demons,
or only ontic errors?

The latter at least dodge
our fear of design; after all
the night sky is not a latchkey afternoon
and the distance to Orion
not that indifferent dyad who never
applauded enough. Those with nothing
                                know:
patterns erupt from us,
but not the shadow sculptures
of Jung's palette swap plasticine
or Campbell's canned journeys;
those Disneyfied scripts elide how we
coax the stars to intimate dread.

It's more that we're viral loads
the void can't suppress, pocking its smile
with dramas like tender sores
so Andromeda remains a maiden
and space remembers to be black.

THE GHOST OF HANA KIMURA

"Frateretto calls me; and tells me Nero
is an angler in the lake of darkness."

I met this ghost on Tinder
after switching settings to the dead,
                      seeking solace
in cavewomen and a floating yokai
                      head, indifferently
swiping right on blood countesses,
                      La Llorona,
catfishing will-o'-the-wisps, Arthur
                      Miller's ex-wife,
an ectoplasmic Tuesday Weld and other
                      restless
types recently divorced from life. Only
                      Hana held
interest, only Hana compelled. At a minute

past moth-pierced midnight,
the point-blank, actual, Instagrammable
                      ghost

of that crowd-murdered wrestler
                        manifested
at the foot of my bed, eyes hollow with
                        hindsight,
haggard and whelmed by a thousand
                        frank opinions
suffered in posthumous limelight.
Death had not mended
Hana's slashed arms; her purple hair
                        had faded
so prettily I almost sneezed. I extended

the canned highball in my hand,
recalling the kitchen where she'd really
                        died
in a fire of furious impropriety—
                        unterraced
rage rupturing the anodyne air
between her and that witless,
                        embarrassed
comedian hiding beneath his hat. To
                        forbear
accurate rage at inconsideration, Hana
                        would have had
to be less earnest, less a child of
                        discipline. The nation

saw a competent woman, not tolerating
incompetence, condemned; then a flood
                              of pious
remonstration. Hana's spirit, not hesitating,
now questioned my evocation: what bias
against the living impelled me? What
                              motivation
had I for swiping through suicides to satisfy
myself, subject as I still was to time?
We opened our highballs anyway, the
ghost's gaze

assessing me. My SuperLike had
                            summoned her in rhyme
and I owed her an explanation: as always,
                              raggedly alone,
condemned to this thankless modulation
                              of sentiment
into structure, I called on the dead, true
                              guides to verse.
A swimmer in nocturnal tides, my
                              shadow had its own
shadow, and indiscriminate access to the
                              unmappable
undersides of light, hope and life came as
                              a condition
of the curse. Did she not consider

these aesthetic exertions the
                equivalent of an honest
athletic career, so that in the strict
                karmic calculus
of sacrificed youth, was there not, at
                least, a veneer
of parallel purity, given that I too had
                labored alone
in obscurity, to even less repute,
                however sincere?
Anonymity at last kills as much as
                hate, depraves
the living spirit, making it long for even
                the public
spite of knaves. Then decades

unrecompensed, each laborious line,
                every witticism
all but unread; survival consigned to
                the loveless region
beyond criticism. Must the sovereignty
                of the dead
be separate? Better infamy, I argued,
                than indifference,
stressing that this was not self-pity,
                only sympathy—
but I saw how far this sophistry had
                brought me.

Hana cannily discerned my purpose
                         and, amused, denied
any similar psychology; applauded only

my misguided pride. None of the real dead
had DMed her botched octaves. At the
                         crack of her smile
we embraced, neither of us wanting to
                         be human,
but with no alternative to beta test for a
                         while,
we lacked an exit more compelling than
                         this clutch
of voluptuous muscles. Tender hours
                         unfurled
until the ghost grew thin with dawn, in
                         her eternal prime
finally impersonal, belonging to all the
                         world.

JASON, KING OF THE VAMPIRES

"Is he really Dracula?"

Jason King as proof and success;
as rat-fanged ruffian, summit of his sex,
a velvet vampire avoiding Germanic excess
for fear of domestic scenes
and laborious smartphone texts.

Jason King revived in the present,
immaculately draining peasants,
not like those unpleasant Romantic
                              impostors,
Hollywood junkies on posters
and other sloppily sparkling poseurs.

Jason King as investigative novelist,
smoking-jacketed hedonist, sidling
                              influence,
Jason King as priest and prince.
Jason King who died a long time ago
and has lived ever since.

THE TYRANNOSAUR OF TRADITION

In so many Boomer Dads
a guilt-green Graham Greene
is conscious of meaning.

In so many sclerotic auteurs
an artless anguished old imp
is conscious of philosophy.

These days I lose track
of so many White Dads on podcasts
armored with unease, camping in the heart
of darkness, praising their own
persistence.

The philosopher father is garbed existence
preceding that molten dream: the real flux,
fixed as soon as recalled. Remember
when he left the Grail on the bus
and no one returned it?

That and other ancestral errors
gave glimpses of the hyenic hindbrain.
Affrighted, he compounded
"Human Nature" from scanned
Russian novels, purblind homilies,
atavistic vagaries—terrors vast
as continents catalogued and cast
in marble over storied centuries.

The tyrant alone with his wisdom,
like a rutting turtle, releases a little
                              sound,
surveying farmers of reckless
                              convention,
General Mills Academy of Nationalism,
the I/Thou of IBM's Antikythera gears
grinding out God and God's attendant
                              fears.

All around are children
waiting to be weighted
with moral mathematics,
relieved of what is variable,
each careless reverie
made less bearable,

and each dream
reduced to reason,

each archetype fixed
in its proper place
like each constellation
in its proper season.

The righteous pose across time
like improper featherless dinosaurs
with bald, simian frowns:

twerpy-limbed hulks gormlessly
crapping out pellets
for credulous crowds.

YOUR OTHER BODY

The miserable anxious you
is only a grub chewing
through days to produce
another body, replayable,
extended and anonymous,
its color-corrected collage
always accessible,
never exactly graspable.

Your other body is not
cosmetic proof of expiring
youth, not a suit stitched
in reproof of candid angles.
That's as if a camera only
copied, as if a picture were
taken rather than pieced
like a speck in a mosaic
or a plasmic scrap in some
archaic cell's living wall.

Your outsides instead
are inside you, the sweating skin
butterfly-wing thin, frailer
than the image encasing you.
That's real skin, zoomable,
adjustable. That's what's got you
in so many hands, homes,
laps, phones. That's what's really
outside the solid ghost. The body
was always inside the soul, not
like a chord in a score or a clean
peg in a dirty hole; the body
just blurred in circles, spinning
blades miming a solid sphere whose
surface—but who cares.

Your other body's all there,
tagged, dated, shared,
pinned, starred, hearted,
safe with God in the cloud,
rough drafts and older versions
cached in canopic folders.

Your other body crushes
my immunity, never lies yet
never stoops to promise,
stops short of compelling
an honest unbecoming:

your other body elopes
without me, dry fevers
grip me as it pierces and
pervades me, entices in slices,
sections itself in stories,
enters me daily yet deerlike
evades me, evokes and revokes
hope, at most quotes me, delays
a final succumbing.

THE GENERATIONS OF GRAHAM GREENE

The old model Graham Greenes
(bits of grit in state machines)
cohered like clockwork pearls
in our pockets and admirably
ejected us each morning
from unearned oblivion.

Now these journalistic organs
expire faster by the year,
though the new models
impale details, snap sharper scenes,
vibrate in the hands of Vietnamese teens,
amass our age in orderly albums.

Obsolescent Graham Greenes
await purgatorial pangs, the mass
melting and scouring for grains
of mineral evil. The good of any
Graham, once so solid in our hands

is at last a mist of toxins, only
a distraction. The hard bright
darkness alone circulates,
reincarnates.

THE ACCREDITED GRAVE

Fêted
      fetid
lauded
      lording plodding
plaudited
modern academic

      mediocrity

crafting and clutching
      a single slender
      verse memoir

to bounce back
      bullets

fired from the future

with nothing
      to their name but

a fungal internet of Tweets
    whisper networks

respectable
    rumors
and verified stances.

    No violent attacks
    on unknown forces.

Nothing reduced

    or prostrated before mind.

Subscribe for the comments
    and scrupulous conscience

of our socially judicious
    aging emerging
guilded guilty
    gilded corpse concealed

in a big big
    big big big
big
    blouse.

FACELESS RECOGNITION

Quarantine cave escapees flee
back to the safety of data

in this bar. Basketball player
birthday girl Megumi

is drunk on martinis. Snapchat,

Snow and Meito-
filtered faces arise
mirage-like, comic animations

a TikTok pocketful
of Korean hand dances.

Meg and I back from the clinic,
old dull sun on her pretty lasered
face post-surgery. I'm now running

out of money. Home after,
I close the window on summer,

flies ablaze in twilit August.
Candle smoke rises

from the ruin of cake. Meg sleeps
cleansed, a monument.

The tiny hopping spider,
my only permanent roommate,

crawls from under the curtain.
                          Info-rich
crypts hum a thumb's touch away,
walls of dead selves sucking esteem.

I lift my phone to scan the spider.
Facial recognition fails—

the spider invisible in its armored
anonymous nudity. It cannot be edited

or improved. Nightly it patrols alone
across that blank Antarctic ceiling.
It is not dead

but does not seem to live.
How does it stay the same

from day to day?

CAPITALIST CATECHISM

In the time it took Eve to conceive
the next generation of consumers,
Adam bought back tracts of the garden
with the wealth of nations, subject to
                                inflation.
Now there are rumors, easy to believe,
concerning the general price of a
                                pardon;
at any rate, the more capital is raised,
the easier it will be for the Landlord
to annul that knowledge they could
                                never afford.
The Landlord's credit plan be praised.

SHIBUYA VS AKIHABARA

The absent Olympics
deride your gentrified
existence. The nymphs now
palely bland, mocked up with managers,
photobooth meccas stashed
in attics, no longer lurid.
Guards tend the gates of an
erstwhile curbside world.

I still haven't graduated
from that dirty McDonald's universe
of marker makeup and curling irons
where darkness was a seizure
of beauty, teenage filth, spring's
branches splashed with blossoms,
fizzy as melon soda. Of course it was
                              always
a race for gold; no style can survive
in a zoo forever—just one neighborhood
"respectfully" correcting the other.

Back from Akihabara, Tartarus of maids:
women angular with images, 4D bodies
trailing archived time. Mazy arcades
cloister silent obsessives with headphones.
Holograms sing their harmlessness
while currency is cemetery energy
in that hideous, populous,
ordered Akihabara.

POSTSCRIPT TO BRAUTIGAN

Long suffering
from the community standards
of dullards, subjected to centuries
of holy massacres, knee-deep always
in well-meaning monsters, let us not
                                      press
our impudent virtues too surely
on any tentative minds still early
in the offing. Machines of sarcasm
and frustrated lust, hermetic machines
humming antisocially, machines that
                                      sleep
past noon, occult machines dreaming
of Enochian avenues, conspiratorial
machines hunting flat Earths and
missing moons, machines selling vinyl
and buying CDs, better these or rank
assassin logics, grey viral gunk,
malevolent bronze Madonnas;
if these convene there is still

some hope for the race, but
in nightmares none outpace
that pristine terror—machines
of "loving grace."

ONLY TENTATIVELY DID I CANCEL GRAHAM GREENE

Only tentatively
did I cancel Graham Greene
withdrawing
my remote from the screen
knowing he would return
in fine form
later down the line
of aesthetic time
dug up and dusted off
as nothing is ever mercifully lost
and period piece morals
update themselves in ages
of equal triteness
pinched into being by the outrages
of educated incompetents—
all that is drab and blithe is ever revived.
"From whence do your values derive?"
asked the greyscale Greene
flashing back into being—

"Are they not disguised
childhood prohibitions
resurrected under rebellious-seeming
posturing and only reversed
on the surface?
Is not my image
a spy inside you?
Who is The Third Man
who walks always beside you?"
It's more that they're instincts
which resist engraving
and that slipperiness
is not weakness
much less the filmic
prancing of a licensed jester
privately pragmatic
in the filched finery
of a sanctioned entertainment
or some professional mourner
wailing over the shroud
of a crosshatched life
morose with enjoyment
of mere complexity.
What's pressed on a child
has no especial authority
much less inviolable 'identity'
beyond reproach
or even poaching

but it is lived through
helplessly as a fever.
What's thought trivial
in that wracking
is the real struggle
not tradition
the politics of place
or a dry beringed
Holiness. You rolled
a cardboard boulder
up a stage
in a costume plucked
from a marriage—
bits of Britain
stuck to one
well-traveled shoe—
scenic gravel.
This prosy removal
with its well-heeled
weariness suited you
but now we have no use
for brick and mortar bits
of affairs and divorces
massaged conflicts
and outdated farces.
An aged man's paltry
batteries cannot at
present be replaced.

Haunt instead some
bloodless other awareness
without bright sharpened
colors or instant decisions.
"OK but I can make a martini—
can I still come to your party?"

DISQUALIFIED FROM BEING DISQUALIFIED FROM BEING HUMAN

No longer Norwegian? No longer human.
The hygge couches clutch at expatriates,
apostates from the census. Trad Norway
FaceTimes its fjords, seeking
                                      reassurance.
Is Maja lost, estranged from heaven,
erecting a rickety existence from foiled
                                      corridors,
hazy monsters of memory, space
                                      compressed
from too much transit; is her life
Blake's 7?

Each fresh terminal suggests an identical
expansion of the Actual. All those fictions,
those chartered nations, don't develop,
                                      just sink

into tics. Haruka, like me a third culture kid,
preens through screens for warmth,
                                  pierces
profiles like a crow cracking snails,
                          drops body
shots for another hundred quid, camgirls
all night whenever she feels jailed.

Alone in Rome, Ramon assembles an
                                 article
of aesthetic war. Sailor makes music
in the street, dreams with dogs and strays,
maps magick across her door. At noon
                                    some
forgetful god or devil arrives in time to see
intransigent humanity, strange as green
                                   lightning.
Maja and Sailor and Haruka and Ramon
and no one I know takes anywhere as
                                    home.

Misled by heritage, twenty-seven
                                isolated
Americans build bunkers full of bullets,
bad teeth, small distinctions of status—
the whole apparatus. A broken mirror
flashes enemy facets, breeds a rival
                                    faction.

Hydra's teeth heroes hunker down in
armor,
unfurling virtuous flags. Now it's time
for action. The whole borough bleeds.

The uncertainties of the publicly-certain
cast borders into doubt; error is ever
doubled
by the undoubting. Perhaps a question
of upbringing? Childhood as a licensed
context rests on a ritual, a forced
conscription.
A child must be defined, discouraged
from doubt;
disqualification from childhood is, as
we know,
entry into the human. Call it an infliction.

Each border brings a neighbor, an
opposite,
thus self. But to stand without all
means self
itself sheds borders, becomes a self of
another
order. Outlasting a context is the
gradual coup
of the counterfeit, what becomes the
Real.

Haruka was handed her identity in a cheap
plastic lunchbox. Was this humanity? Or a
                                    chance
to assemble her self from all she could
                                    steal?

Almost everyone from somewhere is
                                    often
no one from anywhere. Anyone who is no
                                    one
from nowhere might be someone, skew-
                                    wise,
like mismatched socks grabbed from the
                                    hotel floor
or ignoring the objectives of the game to
                                    explore
glitches and no clipping zones.
                    Everywhere a busy
unencumbered no one alights on
                        another's time,
exchanges details, falls down drunk on a
                        foreign shore.

Now the trees are a pleasing plastic, the
                                    soil
is a mobile map and phantom monies
                                    batlike
flit about. The Young Turks are old coins

heavy in nylon pockets, and the Old
                              Turks sing
in their fresh resurrection, melodious
                              dramas
streamed by the New Turks. Gold and
                              other old
standards weigh down only the dead. A
                              heedless
electric geography is etched in every
                              head.

Sailor and Maja trade names, tired of
                              nations,
indifferent rites without mints for
                              dime-bright gods.
No raptures, no transports. What are
                              the odds?
Haruka, horny and bored, caught
                              between passports,
renounces the sense of herself beyond
                              senses.
Rootless cosmicists ransack bland
                              certainty
in Singapore. The sarong parties turn
                              Swedenborgian;
"Love is our only autarchy."

What becomes the Actual, pieced from
what is stolen,
cleanses the conscripted child of the certain.
Bunkers are deserted, coins fall from
                                        pockets
and human disqualifies nation—or at least
in the eyes of Haruka Hernandez and the
                                        whole
improperly formatted conspiracy, arising
                                  from itself,
stateless, viral as a mobile game, a dance
                                          craze;
a desire revised from a nameless inner
                                          flame.

ACKNOWLEDGEMENTS AND DEDICATION

This book is for all friends.

A PARTIAL LIST OF SNUGGLY BOOKS

MAY ARMAND BLANC *The Last Rendezvous*
G. ALBERT AURIER *Elsewhere and Other Stories*
CHARLES BARBARA *My Lunatic Asylum*
S. HENRY BERTHOUD *Misanthropic Tales*
LÉON BLOY *The Tarantulas' Parlor and Other Unkind Tales*
ÉLÉMIR BOURGES *The Twilight of the Gods*
CYRIEL BUYSSE *The Aunts*
JAMES CHAMPAGNE *Harlem Smoke*
FÉLICIEN CHAMPSAUR *The Latin Orgy*
BRENDAN CONNELL *Metrophilias*
RAFAELA CONTRERAS *The Turquoise Ring and Other Stories*
ADOLFO COUVE *When I Think of My Missing Head*
QUENTIN S. CRISP *Aiaigasa*
LUCIE DELARUE-MARDRUS *The Last Siren and Other Stories*
LADY DILKE *The Outcast Spirit and Other Stories*
ÉDOUARD DUJARDIN *Hauntings*
BERIT ELLINGSEN *Now We Can See the Moon*
ERCKMANN-CHATRIAN *A Malediction*
ALPHONSE ESQUIROS *The Enchanted Castle*
ENRIQUE GÓMEZ CARRILLO *Sentimental Stories*
DELPHI FABRICE *Flowers of Ether*
DELPHI FABRICE *The Red Sorcerer*
DELPHI FABRICE *The Red Spider*
BENJAMIN GASTINEAU *The Reign of Satan*
EDMOND AND JULES DE GONCOURT *Manette Salomon*
REMY DE GOURMONT *From a Faraway Land*
REMY DE GOURMONT *Morose Vignettes*
GUIDO GOZZANO *Alcina and Other Stories*
GUSTAVE GUICHES *The Modesty of Sodom*
EDWARD HERON-ALLEN *The Complete Shorter Fiction*
EDWARD HERON-ALLEN *Three Ghost-Written Novels*
RHYS HUGHES *Cloud Farming in Wales*
J.-K. HUYSMANS *The Crowds of Lourdes*
J.-K. HUYSMANS *Knapsacks*
COLIN INSOLE *Valerie and Other Stories*
JUSTIN ISIS *Pleasant Tales II*

JULES JANIN *The Dead Donkey and the Guillotined Woman*
GUSTAVE KAHN *The Mad King*
MARIE KRYSINSKA *The Path of Amour*
BERNARD LAZARE *The Mirror of Legends*
BERNARD LAZARE *The Torch-Bearers*
MAURICE LEVEL *The Shadow*
JEAN LORRAIN *Errant Vice*
JEAN LORRAIN *Fards and Poisons*
JEAN LORRAIN *Nightmares of an Ether-Drinker*
GEORGES DE LYS *An Idyll in Sodom*
GEORGES DE LYS *Penthesilea*
ARTHUR MACHEN *N*
ARTHUR MACHEN *Ornaments in Jade*
CAMILLE MAUCLAIR *The Frail Soul and Other Stories*
CATULLE MENDÈS *Bluebirds*
CATULLE MENDÈS *For Reading in the Bath*
CATULLE MENDÈS *Mephistophela*
ÉPHRAÏM MIKHAËL *Halyartes and Other Poems in Prose*
LUIS DE MIRANDA *Who Killed the Poet?*
OCTAVE MIRBEAU *The Death of Balzac*
CHARLES MORICE *Babels, Balloons and Innocent Eyes*
GABRIEL MOUREY *Monada*
DAMIAN MURPHY *Daughters of Apostasy*
KRISTINE ONG MUSLIM *Butterfly Dream*
OSSIT *Ilse*
CHARLES NODIER *Outlaws and Sorrows*
PHILOTHÉE O'NEDDY *The Enchanted Ring*
YARROW PAISLEY *Mendicant City*
GEORGES DE PEYREBRUNE *A Decadent Woman*
HÉLÈNE PICARD *Sabbat*
URSULA PFLUG *Down From*
JEAN PRINTEMPS *Whimsical Tales*
JEREMY REED *When a Girl Loves a Girl*
JEREMY REED *Bad Boys*
ADOLPHE RETTÉ *Misty Thule*
JEAN RICHEPIN *The Bull-Man and the Grasshopper*
DAVID RIX *A Blast of Hunters*
FREDERICK ROLFE (Baron Corvo) *Amico di Sandro*

JASON ROLFE *An Archive of Human Nonsense*
ARNAUD RYKNER *The Last Train*
MARCEL SCHWOB *The Assassins and Other Stories*
MARCEL SCHWOB *Double Heart*
CHRISTIAN HEINRICH SPIESS *The Dwarf of Westerbourg*
BRIAN STABLEFORD (editor) *The Snuggly Satyricon*
BRIAN STABLEFORD (editor) *The Snuggly Satanicon*
BRIAN STABLEFORD *Spirits of the Vasty Deep*
COUNT ERIC STENBOCK *Love, Sleep & Dreams*
COUNT ERIC STENBOCK *Myrtle, Rue & Cypress*
COUNT ERIC STENBOCK *The Shadow of Death*
COUNT ERIC STENBOCK *Studies of Death*
MONTAGUE SUMMERS *The Bride of Christ and Other Fictions*
MONTAGUE SUMMERS *Six Ghost Stories*
ALICE TÉLOT *The Inn of Tears*
GILBERT-AUGUSTIN THIERRY *The Blonde Tress and The Mask*
GILBERT-AUGUSTIN THIERRY *Reincarnation and Redemption*
DOUGLAS THOMPSON *The Fallen West*
TOADHOUSE *Gone Fishing with Samy Rosenstock*
TOADHOUSE *Living and Dying in a Mind Field*
TOADHOUSE *What Makes the Wave Break?*
LÉO TRÉZENIK *The Confession of a Madman*
LÉO TRÉZENIK *Decadent Prose Pieces*
RUGGERO VASARI *Raun*
ILARIE VORONCA *The Confession of a False Soul*
ILARIE VORONCA *The Key to Reality*
JANE DE LA VAUDÈRE *The Demi-Sexes and The Androgynes*
AUGUSTE VILLIERS DE L'ISLE-ADAM *Isis*
RENÉE VIVIEN AND HÉLÈNE DE ZUYLEN DE NYEVELT
 Faustina and Other Stories
RENÉE VIVIEN *Lilith's Legacy*
RENÉE VIVIEN *A Woman Appeared to Me*
ILARIE VORONCA *The Confession of a False Soul*
ILARIE VORONCA *The Key to Reality*
TERESA WILMS MONTT *In the Stillness of Marble*
TERESA WILMS MONTT *Sentimental Doubts*
KAREL VAN DE WOESTIJNE *The Dying Peasant*

www.ingramcontent.com/pod-product-compliance
Lightning Source LLC
Chambersburg PA
CBHW020549080526
44583CB00013B/1061